Trips

HOW

HALLUCINOGENS

WORK

IN YOUR

BRAIN

Trips

HOW

HALLUCINOGENS

WORK

IN YOUR

BRAIN

CHERYL PELLERIN

SACRED DRAWINGS BY R. CRUMB

AND THE ORIGINAL *ZAP COMIX* ARTISTS, INCLUDING
VICTOR MOSCOSO, RICK GRIFFIN, S. CLAY WILSON,
SPAIN RODRIGUEZ, GILBERT SHELTON, ROBERT WILLIAMS,
AND MANY OTHERS...

SCIENCE ILLUSTRATIONS BY ELLEN SEEFELT

SEVEN STORIES PRESS / NEW YORK

In the U.K.:
Turnaround Publisher Services Ltd., Unit 3, Olympia Trading Estate, Coburg Road, Wood Green, London N22 6TZ U.K.

In Canada:
Hushion House, 36 Northline Road, Toronto, Ontario M4B 3E2, Canada

Library of Congress Cataloging-in-Publication Data

Pellerin, Cheryl.
    Trips: how hallucinogens work in your brain / Cheryl Pellerin.
        p.   cm.
    ISBN 1-888363-34-7
    1. Hallucinogenic drugs. 2. Drug abuse. I. Title.
HV5822.H25P45 1996
362.29'4—dc20   96-30368
                                                       CIP

9 8 7 6 5 4 3 2 1

Book design by Cindy LaBreacht

Seven Stories Press
140 Watts Street
New York, NY 10013
http://www.sevenstories.com/

Printed in the U.S.A.

TO
R. CRUMB
the only guy on Earth who could have made my vision for TRIPS
put on its boots and truck on down

TO
DAN SIMON, publisher, Seven Stories Press
for crossing a diamond with a pearl and turning it on the world

AND TO
IDA PELLERIN (hi mom)
ditto
(See, I *told* you I needed all that money to write a book. Now that TRIPS
is at bookstores, maybe people will buy it and I can start paying back
your retirement money. So... now you can return my calls, right mom?
Hello? Heh heh. What a kidder... Mom? Hey mom?)

CREDITS

Sacred drawings, amazing grace: **R. Crumb**. The notion (to write a book): **Philip Moeller, the *Baltimore Sun***. Facilities, poverty gags (I *think* they're gags): **R Kane @ The Reach**. Chronic financing: **Ida Pellerin**. Color copies, comparative religion: **Phoenix Printing–Kambiz Khalaji & Abbas [haji] Sadeghi**. Real money: **The Hertz family: Judy [Pellerin], Terry, MacKenzie & Harris**. Moving & shaking: **Reputation Movers & Patrick Carr**. Will to live: **Cummings the [good] dog, Lao Tzu, Bill Wilson, the blues (electric)**. Drug of choice: **Caffeine (Ersatz Brothers coffee)**. Services above & beyond: **St. Janet Collins**. In-kind contribution & family tech support: **Judy Pellerin Hertz**. Web site design & apostate of Hell: **Joe Backo**. Spiritual guidance: ***Mystery Science Theater 3000***. Mental health services: **Eli Lilly**. Palm Beach poolside editing facility: **Selma & Mickey Zeiger, Ariana Rinaldi, Jason the wonder dog**. Ms read, fact check, graphics, story edit: **David Nichols**. Molecule integrity, commentary: **Richard Glennon**. Ms. read, fact check, hospitality: **Rick Strassman**. Ms. read & psychedelic lore: **Charles Grob**. Saint-like patience: **Stephen Szára**. Transportation: **Saab**. Transcendental auto repair: **Yates Automotive**. Armed response: **Smith & Wesson**. Mind changing: **Stephen Szára, Jonathan Ward, Jon Franklin, Mark Levy, Timothy Leary**. Speaker-to-artists & art continuity: **Victor Moscoso**. Science illustration, true belief: **Ellen Seefelt**.

with special thanks to

The contributing artists. R. Crumb, Victor Moscoso, [Ida Griffin & the estate of] Rick Griffin, Spain Rodriguez, S. Clay Wilson, Robert Williams, Gilbert Shelton, Jay Lynch, art spiegelman, Kim Dietch, H. Vogrin, Jack Jackson, Ralph Reese, Andy Martin, Yossarian, and the estates of Vaughn Bode, Greg Irons, Rory Hayes & Harvey Kurtzman.

The contributing scientists. Stephen Szára, NIDA (ret.); Rick Strassman; Dave Nichols, Purdue University; Richard Glennon, Medical College of Virginia; Katherine Bonson, NIMH; Charles Grob, Harbor/UCLA Medical Center; George Aghajanian, Yale; Steve Peroutka; Mark Geyer, University of California-San Diego; Mark Molliver, Johns Hopkins; George Ricaurte, Johns Hopkins; Geraline Lin, NIDA; Curtis Wright, FDA (ret.); Abram Hoffer; Raphael Mechoulam, Hebrew University-Jerusalem; Ralph Metzner, Green Earth Foundation.

The Seven Stories publishing team. Dan Simon, Jon Gilbert, Mikola De Roo, Cindy LaBreacht.

Intent

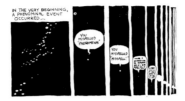

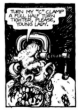
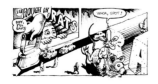

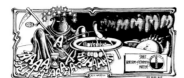
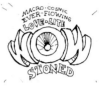
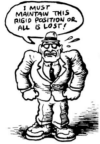

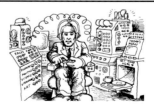
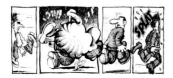

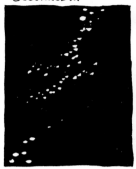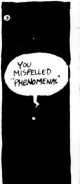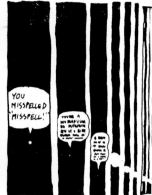

Preface

20th CENTURY, 15 MINUTES 'TIL CLOSING

In a move consistent with his efforts to portray the White House staff as counterculture hippies, this week Newt Gingrich accused Clinton staffers of using drugs. A spokesperson for the White House dismissed the charges by saying, "Man, that's fucked up" [laughter]. Of COURSE they do drugs. Who went through that era of American history and didn't do drugs? You remember the assholes who wouldn't hit a joint? Do you want them running the country? No, of course you don't. You want somebody who cleaned their pipes out with a little blotter.

—Dennis Miller, Dennis Miller Live–HBO, Dec. 9, 1994

IF WE WERE ALL going to hear, right now, everything researchers know for sure about how hallucinogens work in your brain, *Trips* would be so short you'd only have time to say *Tr...*

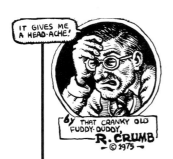

IT GIVES ME A HEAD-ACHE!

by THAT CRANKY OLD FUDDY-DUDDY, R. CRUMB —© 1975 →

I can't tell you how hallucinogens work because no one knows yet. Just like no one really knows *too* much about how the brain works, which is a big part of the whole hallucinogen mystery. A better subtitle for *Trips* would be something like, *How all these really dedicated researchers have spent their careers studying hallucinogens so they can figure out how the brain works, and every year they make a little progress.*

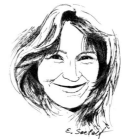

ELLEN SEEFELT

No hard answers, nothing etched in stone. So what you'll read about is how neuroscientists and pharmacologists and medicinal chemists and psychiatrists *think* LSD and other hallucinogens work in the brain. In language I hope everyone can understand. With **cartoons** and **science illustrations**, interviews and research findings, jokes and gags. And every now and then—in chapters describing federal attitudes and actions related to drug enforcement, regulation and public information—**ACTUAL OPINIONS.**

I was a kid in the mid-to-late 1960s and I remember the flow of official 'public information' about psychedelics and other drugs from the Drug Enforcement Administration (DEA), the Food and Drug Administration (FDA) and the National Institute on Drug Abuse (NIDA) or whatever they were called then. Today, a generation later, I know this: no one in *any* federal agency in the 1960s knew enough about LSD and the other hallucinogens even to speculate about their short- or long-term effects on people who took them. And, like actor Tom Laughlin in his 1971 film *Billy Jack*, when I see federal officials using their authority to misrepresent something in the name of public health, "I... just... go... ber*SERK*..."

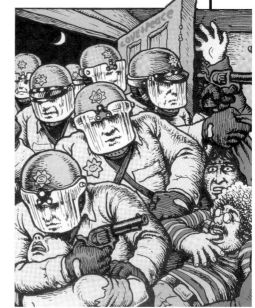

HA. NOT REALLY. BUT IT DOES GENERATE SOME HEAVY OPINIONS, SO YOU WON'T NEED A *LIBRETTO* TO FIGURE OUT WHICH ONES ARE MINE. THAT'S OKAY. YOU GET THE SAME THING, MAYBE A LITTLE LESS IN-YOUR-FACE, IN ANY ARTICLE ON A CONTROVERSIAL TOPIC, WHETHER IT'S PUBLISHED BY DEA, *THE NEW YORK TIMES*, *WIRED* OR THE *JOURNAL OF FISH BIOLOGY*.

In the text I tried to explain any word, phrase or concept I thought might need it. In the interviews I just let the regulators and researchers talk because I thought you'd appreciate the perspectives of people who've studied psychedelics every day for more years than the United Nations has been trying to negotiate a global nuclear arms reduction treaty. I wanted you to hear how they talk about their work, describe the research process, deal with other researchers and think about the drugs they control and investigate and the people who use those drugs.

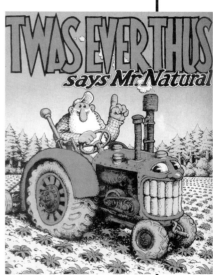

The idea for *Trips* is more than 10 years old. In 1986 I was completing a B.S. degree in science journalism (University of Maryland) and wrote an honors thesis on LSD research. Timothy Leary (1920-1996) gave me a telephone interview and sent an encouraging note when he'd read the paper. Whenever I mentioned the thesis topic, an amazing range of people were interested. And all had equally bad information about hallucinogens. A few years later I realized how many people could use a book that made the news about hallucinogens flowing out of 1990s neuroscience and pharmacology research labs accessible to a general audience.

To write *Trips* I went to technical meetings and seminars on hallucinogen research from 1991 to 1995—to places like Rockville, Maryland; San Diego, California; Lugano-Agno, Switzerland; Victoria, British Columbia; and Washington, D.C. I sat in front rows, IVed coffee, recorded technical presentations and took frantic notes. Over time I arranged interviews with the researchers whose work I

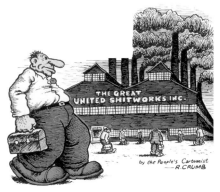

by the People's Cartoonist
—R. CRUMB

was following, and with their cosmic allies and adversaries at federal agencies.

➤ HOWEVER THEY SAY IT, IT MEANS *I DON'T KNOW*

I've never met a hallucinogen researcher who studies hallucinogens just to learn about psychedelic drugs. They're mainly interested in how the brain works. The connection is this: no drug or chemical compound can work in the brain—can affect your brain or body—unless it fits (plugs) into a receptor (picture an organic electrical outlet) on one of the billions of brain cells called neurons. Running through all these brain cells like maniacal bike messengers are chemicals called neurotransmitters that relay messages from the brain all over the body. So at the absolute most basic level, hallucinogens work in the brain because chemically they look a lot like compounds that are already there—compounds the brain makes itself, onsite. That's *why* hallucinogens work in the brain. *How* is another story, but stick around. And hallucinogens look so much like the brain neurotransmitters dopamine, serotonin and norepinephrine that they fit into the same receptors.

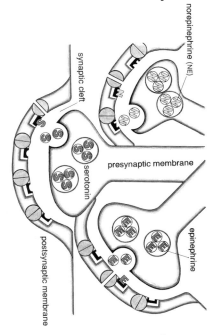

norepinephrine (NE)

synaptic cleft

presynaptic membrane

serotonin

postsynaptic membrane

epinephrine

Researchers figure the more they learn about hallucinogens, the more they'll know about neurotransmitters, neurotransmission and other biochemical mechanisms that regulate brain activities. Why study the brain? Because, at any level beyond basic function and structure, they don't know too much about that, either. And there's nothing wrong with not knowing. Unless, like some medical doctors, you'd rather advertise your practice from a skywriting plane than admit ignorance in public. Hallucinogen researchers don't mind, but they're not big on saying it outright. So in their interviews, when they say an exact effect or mechanism

...isn't fully understood

...has a cause that isn't known

...is still uncertain

...is not yet entirely clear
...needs further study
...is incompletely
understood...

...you'll know what
they're trying to say.

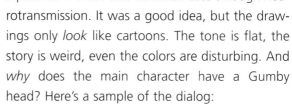

FOR LOTS OF REASONS
— including confusion
— federal agencies,
researchers, publishers,
parents, drug users,
science writers and reporters
have all spread bad information about hallucinogens and other drugs over
the decades. In this decade, organizations like NIDA say they're trying to put
out better drug information in cooler packages. But open the new covers
and instantly you know they're still clueless about how to discuss drugs with
people who actually use them. The writers are way too negative and conde-
scending; they speak too generally, to avoid confusing the audience with
facts; and they use stiff, self-conscious terms that no one familiar with the
drug culture would ever use—*marijuana cigarette, hallucinogen intoxication,*
administering LSD.

One 1994 NIDA student magazine, *If You Change Your Mind,*[1] started
using its own cartoons to explain how brain cells communicate through neurotransmission. It was a good idea, but the draw-
ings only *look* like cartoons. The tone is flat, the
story is weird, even the colors are disturbing. And
why does the main character have a Gumby
head? Here's a sample of the dialog:

Hi...I'm here to talk to you about
drugs and how they can mimic natur-
al processes in the brain. Drugs mimic
natural processes in the brain in a
way that doesn't occur naturally. The
natural process that drugs mimic is
called...

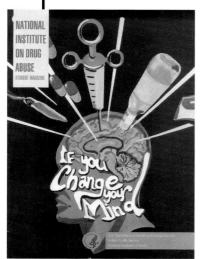

SOURCE: NIDA 1994

...zzzzz ...zzzz zzz z ... huh? Oh sorry.

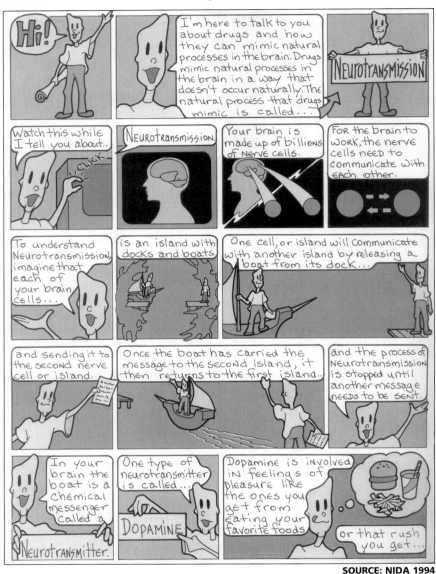

SOURCE: NIDA 1994

CARTOONS DON'T SAY THINGS LIKE THAT. And despite the cartoons and new formats, for *god's* sake don't expect to find humor in any publication or on any Web site funded with federal money. Drugs and brain research and neurochemistry are *way* too serious to laugh at. Aren't they?

Nothing ever stops being serious just because people laugh at it, to para-phrase George Bernard Shaw.[2] And humor's a great way to teach and learn. I know because I write about science for general audiences and I use every tool I can find—pictures, color, jokes, gags. I'd use handcuffs if it'd do me any good. The weird thing is, I have to spend twice as much time researching and studying a science topic to make a joke about it than if I just put facts together for an article or script. And I'm *glad* to do it because an audience appreciates a light touch. Especially when we're dealing with definitely un-light topics like drug addiction and overdose and death.

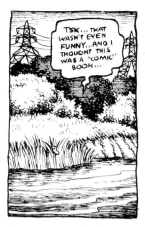

The only drug-related joke ever tolerated in federal circles was Nancy Reagan's screamingly funny **Just Say No** campaign. Well—screamingly ironic. In the 1980s, the former First Lady used her glow-in-the-dark visibility to send America's young people an urgent message. **Just Say No**. It was supposed to be about drugs, but anyone with a brain knew what it really meant—just say no to *thinking: Don't use drugs and don't ask why. Don't examine the issues, don't explore your boundaries. Don't have a debate, take a risk, make your own decisions.*

But the campaign *was* good for *some*thing. Even today, more than 10 years later, people are still cranking out the **Just Say No** parody products. A healthy sign.

On the lacy white useless train of **Just Say No,** soldiers in the fatally flawed War on Drugs locked and loaded and marched off to fight the wrong battle. The whole drug thing starts here, in the brain, not in Colombia, South America.

You can't fight the drug war with guns. Not everyone has a drug problem, but if you do the battle's more like a wrestling match. You and your demons, bare hands, no holds barred. Either way, you use or you don't. The decision's yours and always will be. *Why* is a whole other question.

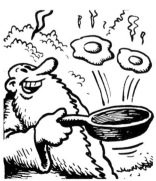

And exactly when will the nonprofit drug warriors figure out, heading into the 21st century, that people need information, not advertising slogans, to make good decisions about whether to use drugs?

**"This is your brain.
This is your brain on drugs.
Any questions?"**

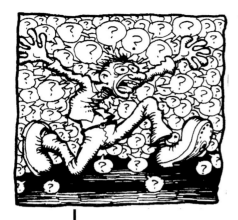

YEAH. I'VE GOT A FEW. Which drugs reduce a brain to breakfast, sunny side up? At what doses? Over how long a time? Taken with what frequency, in what setting, with what preparation? How many eggs do you have to break to put some information into your hip, slick advertising slogans? And—could I have that scrambled with cheese?

I saw this one at a shopping mall where kids hang out on weekends.

 "Reality Check: Between 1991 and 1994, the percentage of 12- to 17-year olds using marijuana nearly doubled. MARIJUANA IS A DRUG. HELP YOUR KIDS UNDERSTAND."

IT WAS NO SURPRISE later when I found out *Reality Check* is part of a new federal public 'education' campaign to—god help us—"counter increases in marijuana use among teenagers that have been occurring since 1991," according to a 1996 press release from Health and Human Services (HHS) Secretary Donna Shalala. The ad campaign and new antidrug booklets like *Keeping Youth Drug Free* are supposed to "help parents sit around the kitchen table and send a clear message to their children that drugs are illegal, dangerous and wrong."

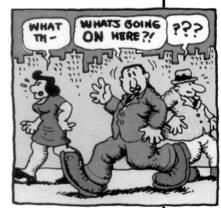

What the hell are they thinking? Anyone who believes 12- to 17-year-olds need help understanding that marijuana's a drug has missed a few of their own regularly scheduled reality checks. Look, most 12- to 17-year olds who smoke marijuana smoke it *because* it's a drug. They don't know much about pharmacology but they know *that*. And what are parents supposed to say? It's hard enough to talk to kids about drugs if you've been there, you're cool and you know *exactly* what's going on with them and with yourself.

For parents—twitching and unconsciously mangling their *Keeping Youth Drug Free* brochures (full of tortured phrases and way too slanted

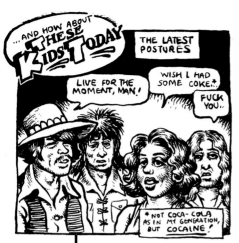

toward use = abuse to even register in kids' brains)—it's impossible. Lots of kids have heard it all already. About the only negative thing kids who already use drugs will believe is that hallucinogens and other drugs are illegal. And the ones who need to have turned ignoring *that* into a science.

Besides, for some 12- to 17-year olds, parents are a big part of the problem. To some teenagers, the world is a nightmare. Sometimes they need a break and drugs are easier to buy than long vacations or 28 days at the Betty Ford Clinic. And there are other reasons. Kids who have mood disorders like depression, for example, and who don't tell anyone or get professional help could try lots of different drugs in an attempt to self-medicate symptoms that can range from hopelessness or anxiety to lethargy or suicidal thoughts. Other kids try drugs because they're curious, or their brains reward them for seeking novelty (see sidebar, next page) or it just looks like fun.

HALLUCINOGEN RESEARCH: WHY BOTHER?

There are as many approaches to hallucinogen research as there are researchers. Why? Because researchers are from different disciplines and have different backgrounds and interests. They're psychiatrists, medicinal chemists, psychopharmacologists, biological psychiatrists, molecular biologists, neurochemists, toxicologists, neurotoxicologists, molecular pharmacologists, biological chemists, neuropharmacologists, ethnopharmacologists and neuropsychopharmacologists. Or you might have a medicinal chemist with a background in endocrinology who spent time in the rain forest with an ethnobotanist—but his *real* interest is molecular pharmacology. You can see how they'd all have different, even multiple perspectives.

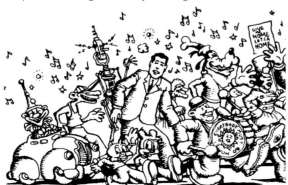

Some researchers focus on where a hallucinogen like LSD goes in the brain to produce its effects. Others do things like compare LSD with other compounds—especially endogenous (made in the body) compounds—that work at the same brain sites as LSD; or focus on the behavior of people who take LSD; or compare hallucinogen effects to disorders like schizophrenia; or see how psychotherapy patients respond to

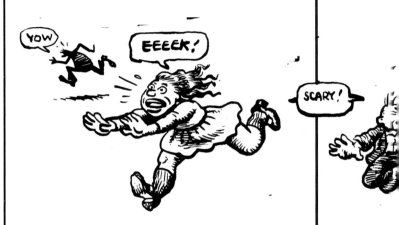

NOVELTY & DRUG SEEKING

In a series of rat studies at the University of Kentucky Center for Prevention Research, Drs. Michael Bardo & Lewis Donohew showed that searching for new experiences may activate the brain's reward system the same way some drugs do. They eliminated the rats' preference for novelty by giving them a drug that blocks brain receptors for dopamine, a neurotransmitter associated with pleasure and drug abuse. Bardo: "We're not saying there's only one biological factor in drug abuse. We're saying there are biologically based individual differences in how rewarding or stimulating people think novelty is. The difference might help explain why sensation-seeking humans might like and use drugs more often than people who don't like novelty." —From an article by Robert Mathias, *NIDA Notes*, a publication of the National Institute on Drug Abuse, July-August 1995

treatment while tripping on LSD; or measure the dimensions of psychedelically altered states of consciousness; or figure out how the body absorbs, metabolizes (breaks down) and excretes LSD. And, like any group of experts in any field, hallucinogen researchers don't always agree with each other's theories, assumptions, approaches, methods, results or findings. The other thing is, researchers sometimes get clear results from experiments but don't always know what the results mean or how they fit with other findings on the same drug. This isn't bad necessarily, it's just the way research works. For years hallucinogen researchers survived regulatory and enforcement terrorists, other federal overseers, disapproving colleagues, a smirking circle of American Medical Association members and a paranoid general public.

They did it because they think it's critical to study hallucinogens and how they work in people. Research psychiatrist and psychopharmacologist Rick Strassman explains why:[3]

⊚ Hallucinogens affect critical aspects of the human mind—mood, thought, will, internal and external perception. Characterizing hallucinogens could help explain mind-brain relationships that lots of people are working to understand—especially in the 1990s, *Decade of the Brain*.*

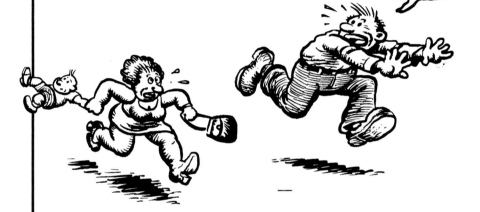

HELP! IT'S GONNA GET ME!!

⊚ Hallucinogens and natural disorders like schizophrenia have common neurochemical features. Understanding these could help scientists learn more about treating mental problems.

⊚ You wouldn't know it from the lack of media attention, but LSD use was pretty constant from the late 1960s to the late 1980s, then rose among high school seniors between 1988 and 1992.

⊚ In early studies, LSD seemed to enhance and shorten the treatment process for some psychotherapy patients.

⊚ Between 13-17 million people in the U.S. have used a hallucinogen at least once (NIDA 1991), and not everyone who uses them has fun. Treating people who abuse LSD or have bad reactions costs money and sucks up dwindling public resources. And there are no safe, selective treatments for bad reactions to hallucinogens.

---

*On July 17, 1990, President Bush proclaimed the 1990s the Decade of the Brain to promote public awareness of the benefits that come from brain research.

SCIENTISTS HAVE LEARNED A LOT about LSD, DMT, mescaline, psilocybin, MDA and MDMA (ecstasy) since the psychedelic '60s, when people blatantly consumed vast quantities of mind-blowing drugs. But research advances are usually reported in the *American Journal of Psychiatry*, *Synapse* or *Molecular Pharmacology*, and not many regular hallucinogen users (past, present, future) subscribe. So lots of people still believe the federal, for-the-moronic-public's-own-good antidrug campaign misrepresentations that originated in the '60s—that LSD breaks chromosomes, causes flashbacks and drives people insane or to suicide. None of that's true. It never was.

LSD DOESN'T BREAK CHROMOSOMES

In his 1994 book *The Natural Mind*,[4] Andrew Weil, M.D., says the *New England Journal of Medicine* first reported that LSD breaks chromosomes in 1967, in a research report by Cohen, Hirshhorn and Frosch. It was called "In Vivo and In Vitro Chromosomal Damage Induced by LSD-25" and said LSD users seemed to have a higher frequency of broken chromosomes in white blood cells, called lymphocytes, than normal people did. In the same issue, an editorial titled "Radiomimetic Effects of LSD" suggested that LSD, like radiation, damaged genetic material. Then there was circumstantial evi-

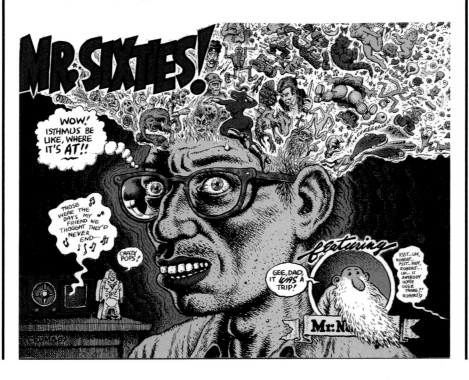

dence: another research team reported that LSD affected the chromosomes of cells growing in test tubes, and a few mothers who had used LSD had deformed babies. It was front-page news and, before the ink was dry, National Institute of Mental Health (NIMH) media people had used the erro-

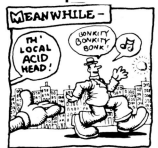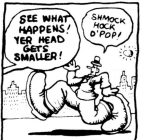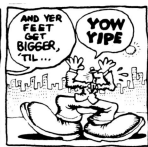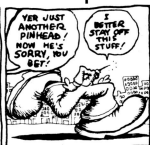

neous results in propaganda campaigns against LSD. But Cohen, Hirshhorn, and Frosch; NIMH and the media ignored some pesky details:

⊚ No one legitimately tested the hypothesis by looking at chromosomes *before* they were exposed to LSD or gave LSD to volunteers in a controlled way and monitored the chromosomes.

⊚ Lots of things break chromosomes—including aspirin, Thorazine and viruses.

⊚ The researchers didn't even try to control for these or any other conditions in the clinical cases they looked at.

⊚ Then there was the problem of tissue-culture studies, because cells that grow in test tubes don't act like cells that grow in the body.

⊚ LSD doses that changed chromosomes in tissue-culture cells used in lab research were lots higher than what living cells get when someone drops acid.

⊚ Everybody has cells with chromosome breaks, but the 1967 study was based on a statistical difference in the *frequency* of breaks in lymphocytes.

⊚ The researchers never mentioned that lymphocytes are among the few cells whose chromosomes anyone can even *see* under a regular microscope.

⊚ Through the whole controversy, no one even showed why it was bad to have lymphocytes with broken chromosomes. It sounds bad, but so does nonfat frozen yogurt.

ACCORDING TO WEIL, all the flaws in the medical arguments against LSD were obvious in 1967. It's okay that the *New England Journal of Medicine* (*NEJM*) published the article, but certain other researchers, NIMH and the press shouldn't have hyped the idea on such thin data. The *Berkeley Barb* and other underground newspapers pointed out the flaws eight months before the *NEJM* admitted it had similar doubts. In 1969, researchers Tijo, Pahnke and Kurland published "LSD and Chromosomes: A Controlled Experiment" in the *Journal of the American Medical Association*. Their work showed no relationship between LSD use and chromosome breaks, and never made the headlines.[5]

"This episode ought to be profoundly embarrassing to journal editors and government scientists," writes Weil, associate director of the Division of Social Perspectives in Medicine at the University of Arizona College of Medicine in Tucson, and president of the Center for Integrative Medicine. "At one stroke it created an irreparable gap between drug users and drug experts," he continues. "Since 1968 I have not met a single hallucinogen user who believes any reports of medical damage associated with drugs, and the use of hallucinogens has never been higher."[6]

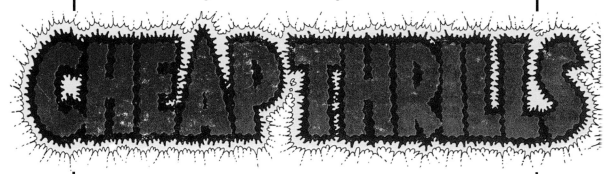

LSD & FLASHBACKS

A drug flashback is supposedly a surprise return of drug-experience elements like visual or auditory distortions long after someone gets high. Doctors like to call them Hallucinogen Persisting Perception Disorders (HPPDs). In the 1960s, some researchers and media people, without the benefit of dropping acid themselves, described a flashback as an unpredictable loss of control caused by persistent or permanent neurological damage that might be linked to suicide. But in November 1995, during the 25th annual meeting of the Society for Neuroscience, research psychologist Shelly Watkins in the Department of Psychology at California State University–Stanislaus showed a closer link between flashbacks/HPPDs and neurotics than between flashbacks and LSD users.

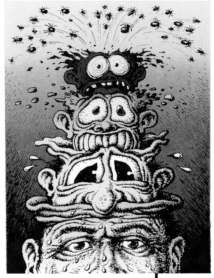

In December 1994, her team distributed 1,000 questionnaires, half to an audience at a Grateful Dead concert and half to people at shopping malls, in classrooms and at work. The survey asked for personal, medical and drug histories, and had a symptom checklist and personality inventory.

Of 360 packets returned, 207 were from people who'd used at least one hallucinogen. Watkins' study of survey responses found that 1 in 5 people who'd used hallucinogens reported having a drug flashback, compared to 1 in 30 who had never used hallucinogens. When asked if they'd had other flashbacks, like from traumatic experiences, 14 percent of hallucinogen users and 10 percent of people who hadn't used hallucinogens said *yes*. Among hallucinogen users, more than half who had flashbacks didn't mind them. The rest were a little, moderately or very bothered. No one said they couldn't function. Hallucinogen users reported more visual symptoms than did nonusers, but only 2 or 3 of 8 symptoms.

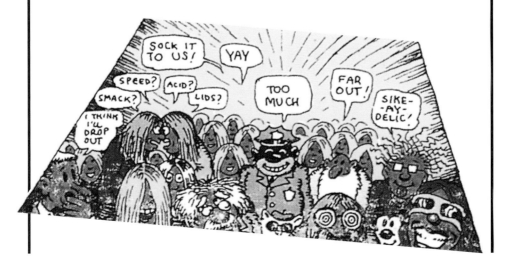

WATKINS' TEAM EVALUATED the relationships between scores on personality inventories that measured neuroticism, extraversion, openness, agreeableness, conscientiousness, HPPD symptoms and flashback reports. Hallucinogen users who scored higher on fantasy and openness were more likely to report 'HPPD symptoms.' Those with higher neuroticism scores tended to report having 'drug flashbacks.' The study strongly suggested that flashbacks aren't too stressful, disabling or uncomfortable, and don't make people lose control. And that higher neuroticism scores on personality inventories might help predict which people would have flashbacks.

GUESS I'M JUST NEUROTIC

> **THE DEA ON FLASHBACKS–1995**
> "Flashbacks are one of the most dangerous side effects of LSD use. They are recurrences of images or effects experienced during a previous LSD administration and they can vary in frequency and duration. Flashbacks can occur spontaneously or can be spurred by the use of other drugs (particularly marijuana or hashish), emotional stress, fatigue, or movement from a light to a dark environment. They can last from a few seconds to several hours. *Ironically, some experienced LSD users do not consider flashbacks an adverse consequence of LSD use and actually enjoy the renewed images as a 'free trip.'* At least they got THAT right.**—**"LSD Use and Effects," A DEA electronic article on the Internet @ http://www.usdoj.gov/dea/pubs/lsd/toc.html, 1995.

SO LSD WORKS IN THE BRAIN. Before we're through you'll understand whether that's good news or bad news—for you. Anyone who's used LSD or other hallucinogens, or who wants to know more about them, has the right to that information. And where do you get agenda-free info about peyote buttons or ecstasy or mushrooms? Mostly you don't. Everyone has biases—friends, parents, police; FDA, NIDA, DEA; reporters and writers, school counselors, pro-drug organizations.

Lots of us tried psychedelics years ago or yesterday and we're *still* trying to figure out what happened. Tomorrow or the next day, someone'll ask another few million of us if we want to try some blotter or ecstasy or mushrooms. Everyone has reasons to say yes *and* no, despite the use = abuse national policy. If 12 million to 17 million people in the United States had tried some *other* substance, and some level number of them had used the same substance every year for the last 25 years, researchers would be all over that thing, pockets crammed with federal dollars. Six kinds of programs would spring up in every federal agency; and some suited-up federal official or outraged citizen would be on a rant about it during every evening newscast.

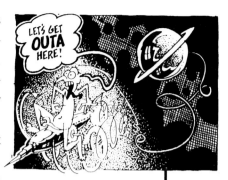

What's so different about psychedelics? That question drives all others in hallucinogen research. Psychedelics do things *to* and *in* and *for* the brain that no one completely understands. Cosmically speaking, they instantly transform everything the brain makes possible—internal and external perception, mood, thought, will, vision, pain, pleasure. We don't know much about the brain, either, but we know this: it makes us unique in the known universe. You'd think an uptight, paranoid species like humans would be more aggressively curious about drugs that pass so easily across the squishy grey line that separates us from everything else.

And before I forget...
This is your brain.   *This* is your brain on drugs

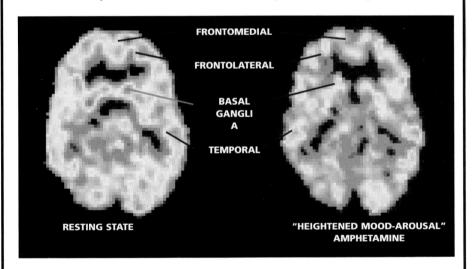

FRONTOMEDIAL

FRONTOLATERAL

BASAL GANGLIA

TEMPORAL

RESTING STATE   "HEIGHTENED MOOD-AROUSAL" AMPHETAMINE

Any questions? You're in the right place.

Cheryl Pellerin
Old Town Alexandria, Virginia
February 1998

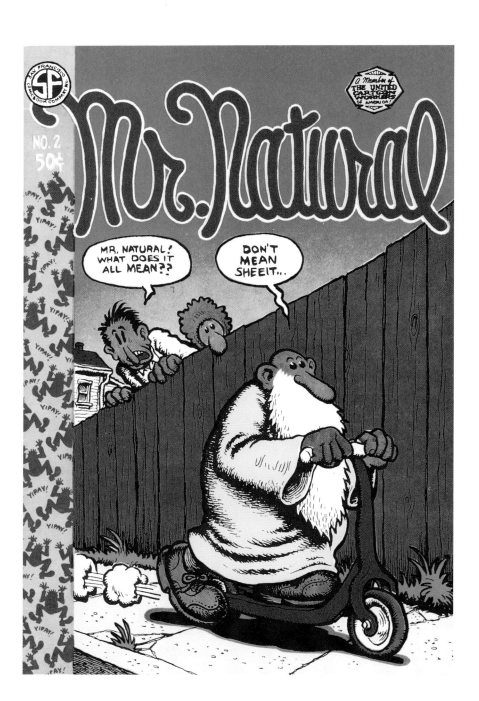

PART I

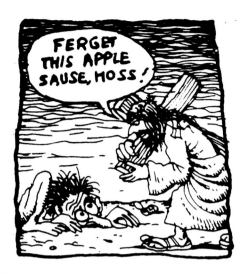

Chapter 1

EVERYBODY WANTS TO GO TO HEAVEN, NOBODY WANTS TO DIE

LSD STUDIES BEGAN mainly with psychotherapy patients, and, in the 1950s and early '60s, researchers used hallucinogens to produce changes of perception, thought and mood that many psychiatrists thought looked a lot like schizophrenia.

Two decades later, in 1962, Congress enacted laws that said researchers had to prove a new drug's safety (it wouldn't kill anyone) and efficacy (it did exactly what they said it'd do) for the condition it was marketed to treat, before it went on the pharmacy shelf. The Food and Drug Administration (FDA) said LSD wasn't even close, and officially made LSD an experimental drug. That meant anyone who wanted to work with LSD had to get FDA permission. By officially making LSD an *experimental* drug, FDA was saying it could only be used for research and never in general psychiatric practice. Now it was impossible for psychiatrists to get legal psychedelics to use in therapy. Some of the best researchers said *Screw this* and walked away.[7] At the same time, some federal officials suggested that doctors who practiced psychedelic therapy brought the LSD crackdown on themselves.

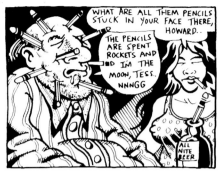
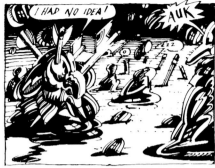

"In a thinly veiled reference to [Timothy] Leary, Drs. Jonathan Cole and Robert Katz of NIMH expressed concern that some investigators 'may have been subject to the deleterious and seductive effects of these agents.'"[8] American Medical Association (AMA) President Roy Grinkler said it was impossible to find investigators who'd work with LSD who weren't already addicts (even though the classic hallucinogens, including LSD, aren't addictive). Grinkler believed public health and safety depended on wiping out all hallucinogen research.[9] Meanwhile, in California, on the East Coast and elsewhere, LSD and other hallucinogens were spreading faster than the Nairobi Ebola virus. Despite FDA limitations and AMA doubts, researchers got federal

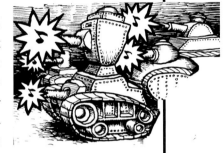

funds to test all kinds of hallucinogens on human volunteers, and more people were exposed to the drugs. Soon, the volunteers started having mighty raucous neighborhood parties. Add this to the growing numbers of private LSD sessions and you had first-round preliminaries to something called the '60s.

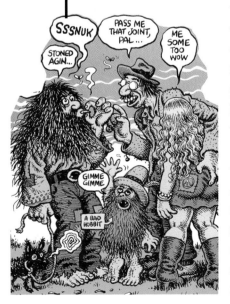

When drug abuse became a national pastime for a visible minority, the medical establishment had a really hard time understanding LSD. It wasn't medicine in the usual sense—it didn't relieve symptoms like coughing or headaches. As drugs not designed to treat specific problems, LSD and other psychedelics were "out of kilter with the basic assumptions of Western medicine."[10]

June, July and August of 1967 was the Summer of Love. LSD, mescaline, MDA, PCP, peyote, DMT, psilocybin, Haight-Ashbury, hippies, headlines, head trips, hassles, heat.[11] The same year, Congress modified the Drug Abuse Control Amendments to make selling LSD a felony and possession a misdemeanor, and shifted enforcement from FDA to the new Bureau of Narcotics and Dangerous Drugs (now DEA).

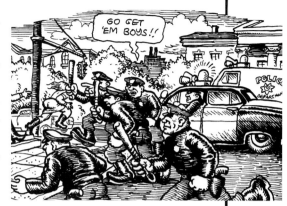

Federal officials were doing to hallucinogens what they'd done to every other drug the dominant culture had no use for—turning the freeway of sacred plants used throughout human history for their spiritual value into a narrow, twisted, badly marked off-ramp called psychedelic drugs. When they realized that compounds isolated from certain plants could change beliefs and behavior, even drive social movements, they panicked and groped for the tear gas and riot gear.

It didn't take them long (probably because they didn't waste time doing lots of pesky research) to announce that psychedelics were so toxic they could kill you and your whole future family. Or worse. And if the drugs didn't get

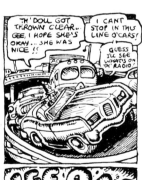

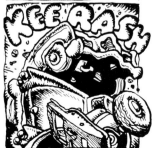

you, the jail time would, because they'd made using, possessing or selling them a crime. Maybe they did it because they feared losing young people to an incomprehensible movement, losing future generations to suicide or insanity and—"maybe any government's worst nightmare—losing control."[12]

In 1970, the Comprehensive Drug Abuse Prevention and Control Act dumped Public Law 639, the Harrison Narcotics Act of 1914, the Marijuana Tax Act of 1937 and every other major drug law passed since the turn of the century into one law commonly known as the Controlled Substances Act (CSA). The CSA cut research in experimental psychoses off at the knees and 'scheduled' all medications and drugs of abuse

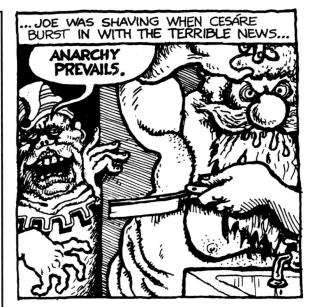

according to *medical utility*, *abuse potential* and *safety of use under medical conditions*. Schedule I was the most restrictive category, for drugs characterized as having no known medical use, high abuse potential and no demonstrated safety under medical supervision.[13] The hallucinogens made Schedule I, but the classification was controversial because earlier studies clearly showed they were safe under medical supervision.[14]

AFTER THAT, U.S. RESEARCHERS had a better chance of replicating Dr. Frankenstein's last life-sciences experiment than of getting federal approval or funding to study hallucinogens in people. They had to turn in their drug supplies. But animal research continued in the U.S. and *some* human studies continued in Europe. Of course, *illegal* LSD field experiments didn't miss a beat.

Twenty years later, in 1990, the tectonic plates of federal drug regulation shifted slightly, the earth rumbled and, for the first time since 1970, FDA approved an application to study DMT in humans.

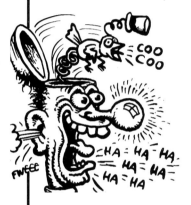

The same year, the National Institute on Drug Abuse agreed to fund the research. Rick Strassman, a psychiatrist then working at the University of New Mexico Medical School in Albuquerque, was the first researcher in a generation to get federal approval and funding to study psychedelics in human volunteers. In a November 1995 personal interview on Victoria on Vancouver Island, British Columbia, Canada, Strassman explained how it all happened.

After years of studying the pineal gland and melatonin, in 1988 he made the leap to hallucinogens by submitting a request to FDA to study MDMA (the mild hallucinogen called ecstasy). This was denied because animal tests showed that MDMA might be neurotoxic, so he put psychedelic research aside and in 1987 submitted a complex melatonin proposal to NIMH. When this came back with a low score, he took off for a month to reassess priorities and on the trip spent time in California with colleagues who, like Strassman, wanted to get clinical psychedelic therapy off the black list. Together they realized that "11 million to 15 million people in the United States had taken a psychedelic compound at least once," Strassman said. "Drugs affect the brain and people abuse drugs and have bad trips. We ought to understand the effects and mechanisms of these drugs in the brain. It was so obvious.

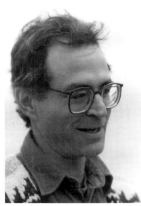

"My colleagues and I figured the most important thing was to be able to treat patients with psychedelics, but not patients the psychedelics might injure," said Strassman. "I wanted to be able to give a group of relatively well-adjusted people DMT and find out what the effects were. I reviewed papers from the late 1960s and early '70s and learned that because of liability concerns some researchers worked only with volunteers who'd taken hallucinogens and planned to continue. That made sense. I didn't want it said that I was turning people into drug abusers. Our study volunteers had to be experienced drug users so they could give informed consent, and they had to plan to continue using them so I couldn't be held respon-

RICK STRASSMAN

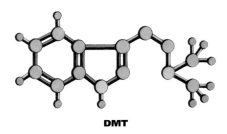

DMT

sible for contributing to a drug abuse problem. They had to be able to handle the drugs and report the drug effects as carefully as they could."

Back in New Mexico, Strassman wrote the hallucinogen research protocol and got it through New Mexico's state reviews and licensing process. In 1989 he started a federal approval process that would last 21 months. It involved the FDA, the Drug Enforcement Administration (DEA) and tons of paperwork, follow-ups, phone calls and bureaucratic firewalking.

Anyone else would have been chewing through their leather straps. Instead, Strassman wrote an article for the *Journal of Psychoactive Drugs*[15] on applying for and getting federal permission to give DMT to human volunteers—the application process, obstacles, solutions, and local and federal issues—in case, he said, "a bus ran me over before I could publish any real data."

Curtis Wright, M.D., deputy director in FDA's Division of Anaesthetic, Critical Care and Addiction Drugs and team leader for addiction products, helped Strassman through the process. In a March 1996 personal interview at the FDA offices in Rockville, Maryland, Wright described

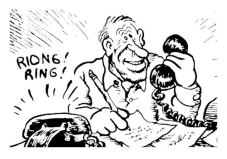

the chronic tension in regulatory agencies between process and outcome:

"In 1989 or 1990, the Pilot Drug Division got specific regulatory permission to depart from traditional agency practices in several ways... One thing that worked was that we went back through every single Investigational New Drug [IND] application that was active but on clinical hold. We found some horrific stuff. For example, Rick Strassman's applica-

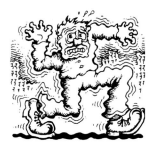

tion. He got caught in a bind we didn't know existed. To get his IND approved he had to demonstrate that his DMT was adequately pure. He didn't have any so he went to DEA and said, *I need a license to make DMT.* They said, *Where's your IND?* He said, *I can't get the IND until I make some DMT.* They said, *You can't make DMT until you get an IND.* So he went back and forth on that one for quite some time before we said, *We'll develop a process by which you can get tentative approval of your IND, then you've got to send us information on the purity of what you're going to make before you administer it to humans.* Things like that were holding people up."

In his article, Strassman shared insights from his excellent adventure: "What can one learn from this at-times-Kafkaesque process? First, with perseverance it's possible to acquire permission to conduct human research with a hallucinogen, in this case DMT. Second, personal contact—primarily by phone and carefully followed-up mailings—are the best ways to keep the process moving forward. Such contact is required, especially to convince FDA, DEA and, at times, the National Institute on Drug Abuse (NIDA) to speak with each other on the researcher's behalf. Third, a simple, scientifically well-reasoned approach with in-house [NIDA] approval is essential, and outside funding is very important. Fourth, a close collaborative relationship with someone who can manufacture hallucinogens may be necessary. If they [already] make the drug, pharmaceutical companies might be inclined. [But] it's better to have a first-class medicinal chemist with a university affiliation.

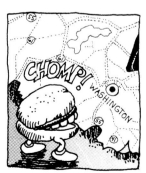

"For researchers interested in studying the use of hallucinogens to enhance the psychotherapeutic or creative process, I believe the same approach, tedious and plodding as it is, might be similarly applied."

AS YOU'RE READING you might notice that some molecular structures for the same drugs are drawn differently. The example below is psilocybin:

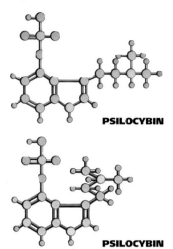

PSILOCYBIN

PSILOCYBIN

According to medicinal chemist Richard Glennon of the Medical College of Virginia in Richmond, molecular structures are flexible and certain bonds can rotate in space. That's called conformational flexibility. Here's an analogy: When you stand, your feet point forward, but you can make your toes point toward or away from each other— these are less preferred conformations. Other conformations are high-energy and unlikely to exist. Like if one foot points forward and the other backward. Unless something's gone horribly wrong, that's an unlikely conformation. In this book, to most effectively show molecular differences and similarities—and because it's such a pain to draw 3-dimensional structures on 2-dimensional pages—the structures are drawn in unlikely conformations. Because they're artistic representations of hallucinogens, we don't care if they're conformationally exact. But to a scientist, Dr. Glennon assures us, they are painful to behold.

LIKE A NEWLY OILED tin man easing out of rusty disuse, in 1990 hallu-cinogen research took a few clanking steps onto the Yellow Brick Road. Investigators have made some progress in the years since 1991, but it's still a long, hard way to Oz.

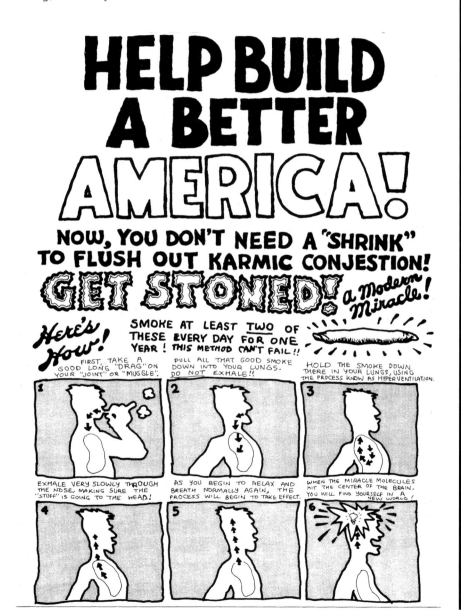

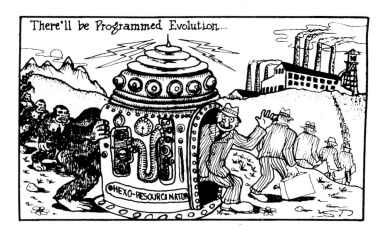

There'll be Programmed Evolution...

Chapter 2

JUST THINK OF IT AS EVOLUTION IN ACTION[16]

Chemistry is applied theology.

—Augustus Owsley Stanley III

INTOXICATION COMES FROM a Latin word meaning *to poison*, but the desire to alter consciousness started *way* before there was language. It wasn't a cure for boredom or the result of satanic intervention. It probably wouldn't have happened at all if every poison plant in the jungle already had a little warning label from the Surgeon General's office. But, as Dr. Ron Siegel wrote in *Intoxication: Life in Pursuit of Artificial Paradise*, all species must have been under constant evolutionary pressure to develop protection against true toxins.[17] They did it by looking for ways to alter consciousness.

People who disapprove of things like intoxication and altering consciousness can probably think of other ways to save a species from obliteration by toxins. But it's the end of the 20th century and 2.5 billion members of *this* species make it hard to argue with success. As James Dunnigan says in *How to Make War*, "If it's stupid but it works, it's not stupid."[18]

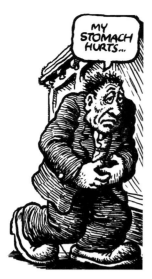

Intoxication can produce sensory and physiological disturbances that cause people and animals to physically reject certain solids or liquids. That's right—heave their guts. But recognizing bitter tastes that led to roiling guts and unspeakable biological disturbances may have taught them to avoid certain plants—a good warning system for the early effects of toxins. Heaving guts or learning to hate certain tastes could have been an advantage for animals or early humans who routinely dined in toxicologically risky places.[19]

Even before advanced medical technology, doctors were pretty good at spotting a poison. You swallowed it. You died. It was toxic. Now, thanks to molecular biology, scientists often know in advance if an intoxicant is also toxic. But so many details of brain and body function are still mysterious enough that even today doctors don't always know how or why things are toxic, even a zillion years after hallucinogenic plants started leaving trails across the visual field of human experience.

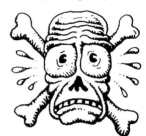

◤ ALKALOIDS

Like all plants, hallucinogenic plants have hundreds of chemical components. Fresh hallucinogenic plants are more than 90 percent cellulose (skeleton equivalent) and water (blood equivalent). Carbohydrates like starches and sugars, proteins, fats, mineral salts and pigments make up a few more percent. But less than 1 percent has anything to do with their mind-blowing effects.

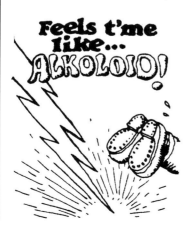

This less-than-1 percent of stuff that affects mind, emotions, perception and consciousness are chemicals now called alkaloids. They aren't built like other plant parts, and researchers still don't know what alkaloids *do* in plants or why some plants have 'em and others don't. In the lab, plant chemists (*phyto*chemists—from the Latin word for plant) separate psychoactive components from the plant and purify them. Now they can synthesize the parts and make their own psychoactive compounds at will.

In 1806, pharmacist Friedrich Serturner made the first psychoactive component in pure form—morphine, from the opium poppy. In 1817 he called

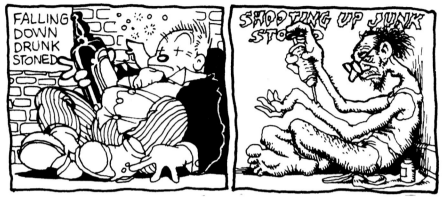

morphine a salt-forming *alkali,* and chemists ever since have called elements with the same properties alkaloids.

Chemically, alkaloids are nitrogen-containing plant products like strychnine and cocaine that have big physiological effects in small amounts. They've been the basis of crude drugs and poisons across history and cultures. Researchers who study human use of primitive drugs are ethnopharmacologists, and they come from almost every corner of science—cultural anthropology, linguistics, history, botany, zoology, chemistry, pharmacology, toxicology and medicine.[20] This broad sweep of the planet's 3-billion-year-old drug scene tends to put a narrow view of drugs into cultural and historical perspective.

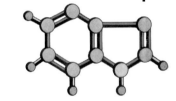

INDOLE RING

Today, ethnopharmacologists and others know the most important botanical hallucinogens look a lot like biologically active compounds in the brain. Some of the compounds Albert Hofmann, chemist at the Sandoz company in Basel, Switzerland, isolated are indole-tryptamine derivatives that look chemically like serotonin, a major brain chemical that may regulate things like mood and appetite.

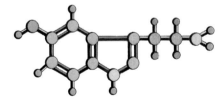

SEROTONIN (5-HT)

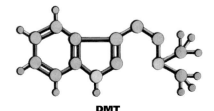

DMT

FORWARD, INTO THE PAST[21]

The Paleolithic Age was a cultural period that started with the earliest chipped stone tools, about 750,000 years ago, and lasted until the Mesolithic Age, 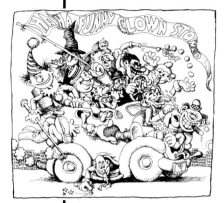 about 15,000 years ago. Many experts agree that, near the end of the Paleolithic, migrant nomads must have traveled from Siberia to the Americas through the Bering Strait, which at that time— lucky for them—was probably a continuous land bridge instead of water. The nomads had what's now called a strong shamanistic tradition based on the ritualistic use of *Amanita muscaria*—a hallucinogenic mushroom called fly agaric because it was first used to kill flies.

CLASSICAL HALLUCINOGENS

FLY AGARIC In tribal societies, a shaman is psychotherapist, clergyman and doctor.[22] Shamans were the earliest medicine men and women and a tribe's link to the spirit world.[23] Hallucinogenic plants and other trance-inducers were their toll-free hotline to the gods. Ceremonies began when a shaman took the magic drink or snuff and went into a trance. Tribe members gathered around to sing, dance and clap their hands. The shaman's trance deepened. The tribe members shook; their arms and bodies vibrated. As most high-dose hallucinogen users can confirm, tripping on powerful psychedelics can put people face to face with overwhelming visions and experiences. You can see how, in nonliterate people, such experiences tended to strengthen their belief in the spirit world.[24]

Shamanism based on *Amanita* started in prehistoric times, before the first nomadic tribes surfaced in the Americas. It might even have been Soma, a sacred hallucinogenic mushroom that the tribes of ancient India "considered a gift of the gods if not the gods themselves."[25] This 'god-narcotic' was introduced 3,500 years ago by Aryan invaders who worshipped the hallucinogen and drank its extract during sacred rites.[26]

When the immigrants finally stumbled onto the American continent and approached the equator, they found more plants than anyone had *ever* seen. Thanks to the warm, humid weather, the density of plant species here that had psychotropic (mind-changing) properties was higher—no pun—than anywhere else on the planet. Of the botanical hallucinogens used in shamanistic rituals and for healing, almost 100 kinds came from the Americas. Only about 12 came from Old World cultures. So it's no accident that even today some South American Indians know more than the gods about growing, harvesting and using botanical hallucinogens.[27]

Investigators in the Sahara Desert found ancient mushroom paintings that a group of pre-Neolithic Early Gatherers in Algeria's Tassili region may have made between 7,000 and 9,000 years ago. The paintings could represent the first documented ritual use of hallucinogenic mushrooms by Paleolithic people. And, investigators at Chile's San Pedro de Acatama archaeological site found the remains of hallucinogenic snuff and paraphernalia dating from 320 to 910 A.D.

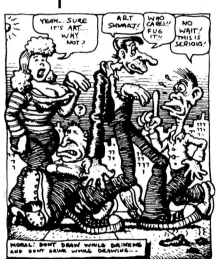

Shamans and others used hallucinogens mainly to channel declarations of divine will—like translators at the United Nations—from the gods to the spiritually challenged tribal flatlanders. An example might have been the Oracle of Delphi. Oracles were divine prophecies, usually told as stories where each person, place and thing symbolized some spiritual idea or moral principle and had to be torturously interpreted. The Oracle of Delphi in ancient Greece was at one of the temples of Apollo—the mythological god of the sun, prophecy, music, medicine and poetry. At the Oracle, a spiritual guide went into a trance, breathed a vapor—maybe smoke from hallucinogenic henbane seeds—that came from cracks in the rocks, and delivered messages from Apollo to knowledge seekers.[28]

Something like 9,000 years later, in another temple—this one built to honor Sandoz and the gods of chemistry—a hard-working researcher named

Albert Hofmann breathed a vapor and in time became a spiritual guide. Today, half a century later, the message he delivered is *still* being torturously interpreted. With no resolution in sight.

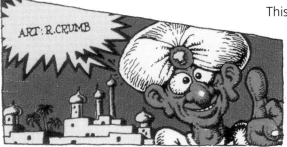

This is true mainly because:

1. Citizens of late 20th century industrial cultures are fragmented and paranoid about religious and spiritual practices unknown to them, although segments of these populations readily believe in things like the Psychic Hotline.

2. If that isn't enough, their very ignorance has led to a great misunderstanding of drugs and their spiritual application and effects.

3. Even scientists only know some very tiny percentage of what could be known about a) drugs and how they work, and b) the brain and how it works. But they're working on it and they know lots more than they used to.

HEAD TRIPS

So if you want to know how LSD and other psychedelics work, you have to know a little about the brain. We'll do it the way people say Einstein liked to—by making things as simple as possible, but not simpler. And thanks to magnetic resonance imaging (MRI), positron emission tomography (PET)

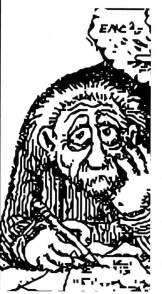

scans and molecular biology, there's a lot more to talk about than there used to be.

You don't have to be dead
NONINVASIVE BRAIN IMAGING

In the 1970s, computers made it possible for researchers to pass x-rays through the brain, then process them into a single whole-brain image. These were the first direct pictures of brain anatomy in living humans. Today there are lots of ways to watch real-time activity in your brain, and you don't even have to be dead. Researchers use a variety of these images to understand the links between brain structure/function and behavior, which could revolutionize brain disorder diagnosis and treatment.[29]

Major imaging techniques are positro emission tomography (PET), single-photon-emission computed tomography (SPECT) and functional magnetic resonance imaging (fMRI). They all detect biological activity in the brain by measuring changes in neurochemical patterns, blood flow, or glucose use. PET and SPECT measure activity in the brain; MRI detects the underlying structure; fMRI does both. Merging images that show brain activity *and* structure produces a hybrid image that lets scientists target the location of specific brain activity. So if someone on a hallucinogenic dose of LSD is on the fMRI machine at the same time (bummer), researchers could get information about what's happening in the brain during the visual distortions, and where it's happening.[30]

PET

POSITRON EMISSION TOMOGRAPHY (PET) scanning lets researchers see real-time chemical processes of cell function in the brain. PET studies use a machine called a cyclotron to label drugs or other chemical compounds like glucose with small amounts of radioactivity. The labeled compound, called a radiotracer, is injected into the bloodstream and taken

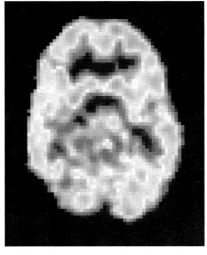

up into the brain. At the subatomic level, the radiotracer emits positrons. These collide with electrons to produce photons, which are detected by crystal rings that make up the PET scanner. When photons hit the crystals they give off light, which a computer converts to 2- or 3-dimensional images that show where the radioactive compound is in the brain. Scientists use radiolabeled water or glucose with PET to show how different experimental conditions activate certain parts of the brain. They also use minute amounts of radiolabeled drugs with PET to show changes in neurochemical systems and track the brain's response to chronic drug abuse, withdrawal, and drug craving.

SPECT

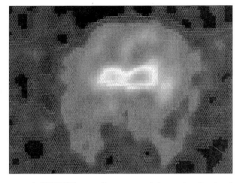

SPECT, LIKE PET, uses radioactive tracers and a scanner to record data that a computer turns into 2- or 3-dimensional images of active brain regions. PET tracers can monitor more kinds of brain activity than SPECT tracers can, but SPECT tracers last longer so labs don't need on-site cyclotrons to produce them, and SPECT studies need less technical and medical staff support. PET's more versatile than SPECT and produces more detailed, higher-resolution images, especially of deep brain structures. But SPECT is much less expensive and can handle lots of the same research questions.

MRI, fMRI

MRI WORKS because the nucleus of an atom has a magnetic property. The property's called nuclear magnetic resonance (NMR) and that's what the technology used to be called. But the word nuclear scares people, even though it has nothing to do with nuclear radiation, so now it's MRI, not NMR.[31] In the MRI scanner, a huge magnet creates a magnetic field around

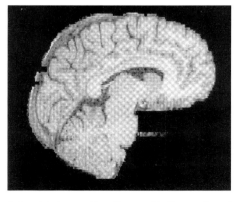

a patient's head. The field is so powerful it causes atomic nuclei in the patient's body to line up parallel to the field. A coil in the imager jars the magnetic nuclei with radio waves, and molecules exposed to an intense magnetic field absorb certain radio wave frequencies.

This magnetic resonance creates a faint radio signal that a computer amplifies and translates into high-quality 2- or 3-dimensional images of brain structures. MRI produces detailed images of surface and deep brain structures and detects tiny structural changes over time. Researchers later found ways to use MRI to image brain activity in progress.

Because blood has magnetic properties, functional MRI (fMRI) lets them see and film real-time images by tracking how blood flow, as a measure of brain activity changes in response to experimental stimuli.

IN 1791, ITALIAN ANATOMIST Luigi Galvani used severed frog legs to show that electricity is a force in the body. His experiments revealed it was possible to use electrical currents to control a frog's motor nerves. Life and electricity—the notion that they're linked—attracted public attention and inspired a young woman named Mary Wollstonecraft Shelley to write a book called *Frankenstein,* published in

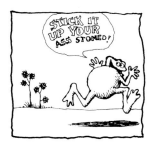

1818. In 1838, Czech physiologist Jan Purkinje figured out that nerve cells, like other cells, had a nucleus—a complex, spherical body in a living cell that holds the cell's DNA and controls cell metabolism, growth and reproduction.

BUT PURKINJE REALIZED neurons had something other cells didn't—sets of fibers that sprouted from the nucleus, later called axons and dendrites. Galvani didn't have the technology to measure the body's really small electrical currents, but in 1850, German physiologist Emil Du Bois-Reymond clocked electrical pulses that blew from brain cell to brain cell at 200 miles an hour. In 1870, Italian histologist (someone who studies tissues and cells) Camillo Golgi stained cells with silver salts, producing much more cell detail than organic dyes did.

The new staining technique helped him see two things— that the central nervous system had billions of neurons, and that

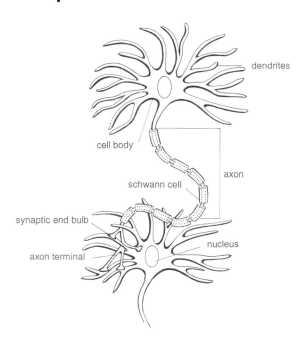

dendrites

cell body

schwann cell

axon

synaptic end bulb

nucleus

axon terminal

German anatomist Heinrich Waldeyer was right when he said the nervous system was made of separate cells and extensions that approached each other but didn't connect. Now Golgi could see that nerve cell fibers left tiny gaps called synapses. He also figured out that the brain sent information to motor nerves, and that sensory nerves traveled to the brain for analysis.

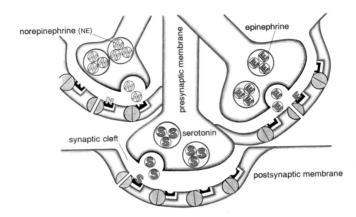

IN THE EARLY 1900s, physiologists Edgar Adrian, Herbert Gasser and Joseph Erlanger discovered that electrical pulses caused neurons to release chemicals (neurotransmitters) that carried messages across synaptic gaps and passed them on to other brain cells. They calculated that it took a neuron one thousandth of a second to recharge after firing. They were right, but the concept of chemical neurotransmission wasn't accepted as a universal process until around 1950.[32] These and other discoveries are the foundation of bleeding-edge neuroscience heading into the 21st century.

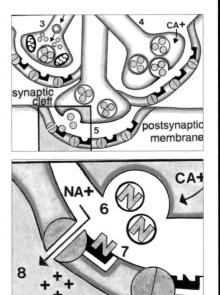

▶ EVERYTHING YOU NEED TO KNOW ABOUT THE BRAIN TO UNDERSTAND HALLUCINOGENS. AND LESS.

HERE'S HOW STUFF LIKE LSD ends up in the brain, starting at the mouth. You swallow a drug. It goes to your stomach and intestinal tract. Some drugs, like LSD, start metabolizing right there. The unmetabolized stuff diffuses through the intestine into the bloodstream. From the bloodstream, a drug can affect any organ system that'll let it in. Like the brain, or the liver.

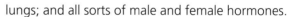

Now the circulatory system carries drug molecules to major organ systems. First, they go to the liver for industrial-strength metabolism. After the skin, the liver is the body's largest organ. It filters circulating blood to extract and destroy toxins. It secretes bile into the small intestine to help digest and absorb fats. It stores vitamins, synthesizes cholesterol, metabolizes or stores sugars, assembles amino acids into proteins and regulates blood clotting.

In the reproductive system, if a female drug user is pregnant and the drug can cross the placenta, it can end up in the baby's blood. Nursing babies can absorb some drugs from breast milk. On the way to the brain, a drug can affect heart rate, pulse rate and blood pressure; breathing and the lungs; and all sorts of male and female hormones.

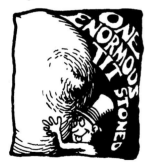

Meanwhile, back at the central nervous system, anything that gets into the brain has to make it through the brain's own system of chemical protection, mainly the blood-brain barrier. Tight cell-wall junctions and a layer of star-shaped cells called astrocytes around the blood vessel keep big or electrically charged molecules from passing into the brain from the blood. Special carriers escort nutrient molecules across the blood-brain barrier. But small neutral molecules like LSD's or THC's can get through without a backstage pass.[33]

For *most* people, the brain is the center of human consciousness. It's so complex that no one knows how it works as a system. Over time, for one reason or another, neuroscientists have opened enough skulls to know what happens in most parts of the brain, if not how or why it happens.

Neuroscientists describe the brain in terms of cortexes and lobes and areas and fields and centers. We don't need to know all that. But we *do* need to know about a few of the brain's working parts, and a *whole* lot more about how brain cells and ion channels and neurochemicals and synaptic gaps and receptors become ecstasy and terror and screaming laughter and awe. Together, these processes are the brain's voice and language, and the reason psychedelics aren't like other drugs.

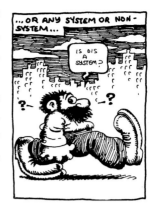

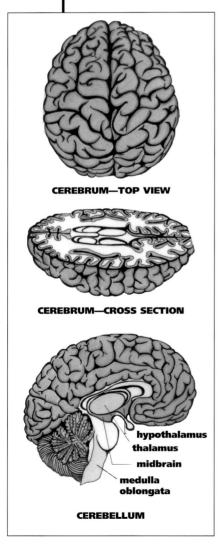

CEREBRUM—TOP VIEW

CEREBRUM—CROSS SECTION

hypothalamus
thalamus
midbrain
medulla
oblongata

CEREBELLUM

THE CEREBRUM COMES in two hemispheres—left and right—and covers most of the brain. Its main job is consciousness, which includes higher mental processes like interpreting sensory output and initiating voluntary muscle movement. The cerebrum's outer layer is the cerebral cortex, the most instantly recognizable brain feature. Those slimy gray convolutions, curving over the midbrain and cerebellum like the worst perm anybody *ever* had, are packed with 10 billion brain cells called neurons.

The cerebellum,[34] under all the grayish stuff, comes in two lobes and controls balance and complex muscular movements. The medulla oblongata and the hypothalamus control internal organs. The thalamus gets sensory impulses from all parts of the body and channels them to the cerebrum. But if you want to understand psychedelics, the most important elements are neurons, neurotransmitters and receptors.

The brain has two kinds of cells. Neurons (15 percent of brain cells) are supposed to be the main information carriers, the brain's basic working units.[35] The other 85 percent are different kinds of glial cells that may be a kind of support cell for neurons, but evidence for that or any other exact function is thin.[36] So who knows what they really do?

THE NEURON HAS A CELL BODY with a standard nucleus and a wild fringe of offshoots called dendrites (from the Greek word for tree branches), typically 10,000 or more. Also extending from the cell body is a long conducting fiber called an axon that (probably) branches into smaller axons before it ends. The nerve endings form synapses with other neurons. These are specialized contact zones—gaps actually—between the end of one neuron (*presynaptic neuron*) and the receptors on the dendrites of another (*post*synaptic neuron). Messengers that carry nerve impulses across the gap are neurotransmitters.

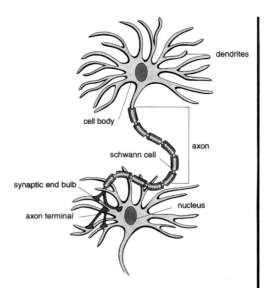

NEUROTRANSMITTERS

Until the 1970s, researchers had only studied about five neurotransmitters in detail. Even now, in the 1990s, lots of antidepressants and other psychoactive (mood changing) drugs psychiatrists prescribe are based on the same five neurotransmitters, including acetylcholine, norepinephrine, dopamine and serotonin. Now scientists know there are at least 50, maybe 100 or more,[37] different neurotransmitters carrying messages around the brain, each the potential basis of whole families of new drugs to treat things like depression, schizophrenia, eating disorders and more.

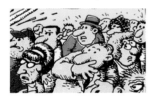

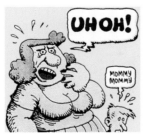

Learning enough about neurotransmitters to create new drugs takes what everything always takes—money, brains, money, time and more money. And like everything else associated with the brain, the following roles and actions of neurotransmitters are suspected, not etched in stone.

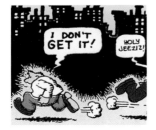

SEROTONIN

Chemically, serotonin is 5-hydroxytryptamine, or 5-HT. Like most neurotransmitters, it's a simple chemical with complex pharmacology. The average adult only has about 10 mg. In the intestinal wall, serotonin makes sure the gastrointestinal tract can move when it needs to. It works in blood vessels all over the body (including the brain) so they can contract when *they* need to. And in the brain it helps regulate sleep, memory, learning, body temperature, mood, behavior (including sex), cardio-vascular function, the endocrine system and maybe pain perception.

Serotonin is involved in the body's reaction to mood-changing chemicals like LSD and some of the most commonly prescribed antidepressants. LSD

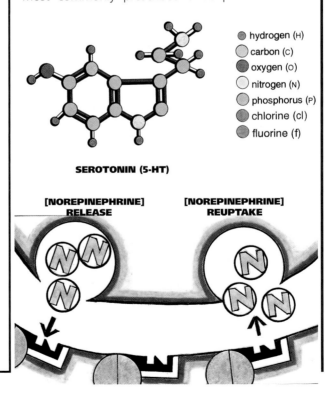

hydrogen (H)
carbon (C)
oxygen (O)
nitrogen (N)
phosphorus (P)
chlorine (Cl)
fluorine (F)

SEROTONIN (5-HT)

[NOREPINEPHRINE] RELEASE

[NOREPINEPHRINE] REUPTAKE

and serotonin-releasing drugs like fenfluramine (used in appetite control)—which cause synaptic vesicles to release more serotonin than normal— work at serotonin neurons to raise serotonin levels in the brain. Prozac, one of a growing number of selective serotonin reuptake inhibitors (SSRIs), acts at serotonin reuptake carrier structures to block the neuron's recycling of serotonin and raise serotonin levels *that* way. More about LSD and antidepressants later.

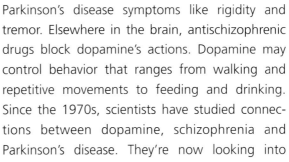

- ● hydrogen (H)
- ○ carbon (c)
- ● oxygen (o)
- ○ nitrogen (N)
- ● phosphorus (P)
- ● chlorine (cl)
- ● fluorine (f)

LSD

DOPAMINE

Dopamine was discovered as a neurotransmitter in 1958 in the brain's corpus striatum, which regulates body movement. Destroying dopamine neu-

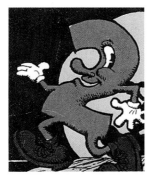

rons here causes Parkinson's disease symptoms like rigidity and tremor. Elsewhere in the brain, antischizophrenic drugs block dopamine's actions. Dopamine may control behavior that ranges from walking and repetitive movements to feeding and drinking. Since the 1970s, scientists have studied connections between dopamine, schizophrenia and Parkinson's disease. They're now looking into dopamine's role in all kinds of drug abuse and how it might help explain disease, addiction and treatments for both.

NOREPINEPHRINE

Norepinephrine is one of two major catecholamine neurotransmitters. It was characterized in the 1930s as the transmitter used by the autonomic nervous system's sympathetic nerves. These control emergency responses like accelerating the heart, dilating the bronchi and raising blood pressure.

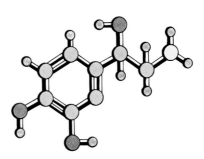

NOREPINEPHRINE

THE BRAIN'S DRUG REWARD SYSTEM

From NIDA Notes, a publication of the NIH National Institute

on Drug Abuse, Sept/Oct 1996

Researchers who want to know which brain structures are involved in the human drug reward system have learned a lot from rat studies. Because brain chemistry is similar in people and rats, investigators think the addiction process might be similar too.

These theoretical human drug reward systems come from animal data to show which areas may be involved in human brain reward systems.

COCAINE-AMPHETAMINES

The cocaine-amphetamine reward system includes dopamine-using brain cells (neurons) in the ventral tegmental area (VTA) that link to the nucleus accumbens and areas like the prefrontal cortex.

OPIATES

The opiate reward system includes the VTA, nucleus accumbens and prefrontal cortex. Opiates also affect the arcuate nucleus, amygdala, locus ceruleus and periaqueductal grey area. All use neurotransmitters that act like heroin and morphine.

ALCOHOL

The alcohol reward system includes the VTA and nucleus accumbens, and affects the cortex, cerebellum, hippocampus, superior and inferior colliculi and amygdala. All use gamma-aminobutyric acid (GABA) as a neurotransmitter.

The VTA and nucleus accumbens are involved in the reward system for all drugs, including alcohol and tobacco, but other mechanisms might be involved for specific drugs.

GABA (GAMMA AMINOBUTYRIC ACID)

GABA has no known function besides working as the brain's most common inhibitory neurotransmitter. That means it slows down neuron firing. Alcohol and benzodiazepine tranquilizers like Valium both work at the GABA receptor.

 The real voice in your head

SYNAPTIC TRANSMISSION

Among people, words and voice and language are bricks in the wall of communication. Not much happens unless people exchange ideas and information, and the same thing's true in the brain. Here, electrical impulses and neurotransmitters and synaptic gaps make it possible for neurons to communicate. Only now it's called neurotransmission, and it's the basis of everything except giving law enforcement officials control over any aspect of the scientific research enterprise.

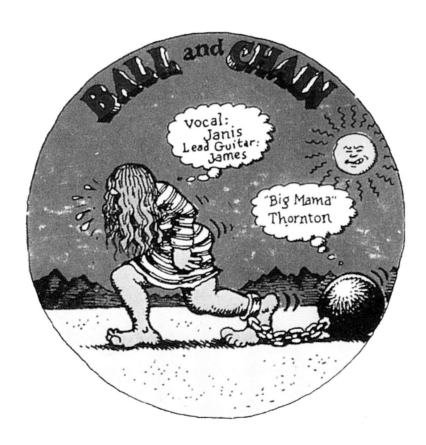

HERE'S HOW NEUROTRANSMISSION WORKS:

1. Something happens. A stimulus! You win the lottery. You take a drug. The stimulus generates a nerve impulse in the dendrite or cell body.

2. The nerve impulse triggers a series of electrochemical waves (I'm skipping a lot of stuff here about sodium and potassium ions, electrical potentials and positive and negative charges—which are why neurotransmitters are called electrochemicals) that hustle down the axon toward the nerve terminal. The cell is firing.

3. Meanwhile, here at the business end of the neuron, enzymes and other stuff use precursor chemicals to build their own neurotransmitters and store them in synaptic vesicles.

4. So here comes the nerve impulse, blasting down the axon. When it hits the nerve terminal, synaptic vesicles fuse with the outer membrane and create temporary openings.

5. When this happens, all their stored neurotransmitters dump out of the presynaptic neuron and into the synaptic gap (I always picture this as watery). Splash!

6. Now the neurotransmitter molecules are in the gap. A couple of things might happen, but let's say they do their main job: they cross the gap like a shotgun blast to the dendrites of the postsynaptic neuron.

7. For neurotransmitters to have any effect on the postsynaptic neuron, they have to be able to bind to specific receptor sites on the dendrite branches. Receptors are the sites of action for any chemical, whether it's endogenous (made in the body) or from Ersatz Bros. Drug Co.* or the local drug dealer.

7A. Each kind of neurotransmitter molecule—serotonin, dopamine or whatever—has its own membrane-protein receptor. A form-fitting organic 'socket' that only recognizes the shape of its own neurotransmitter or something *really* close. This means a couple of things: neurotransmitters only affect neurons that have the right receptors, and neurons with lots of receptors can react more energetically than neurons with just a few receptors.

7B. Another thing about neurotransmitters, they're either excitatory or inhibitory. At the nerve ending the incoming electrical impulse triggers a neurotransmitter release. It diffuses across the gap and binds to a receptor on the

---

*From the wonderful folks who brought you Ersatz Brothers Coffee—Firesign Theatre, *Shoes for Industry*: Disc 1, 1993, CD Columbia C2K 52736. Fans should check out http://www.cs.umd.edu/users/dabe/CDs/Songs/ersatz.bros.coffee. html and other FT links.

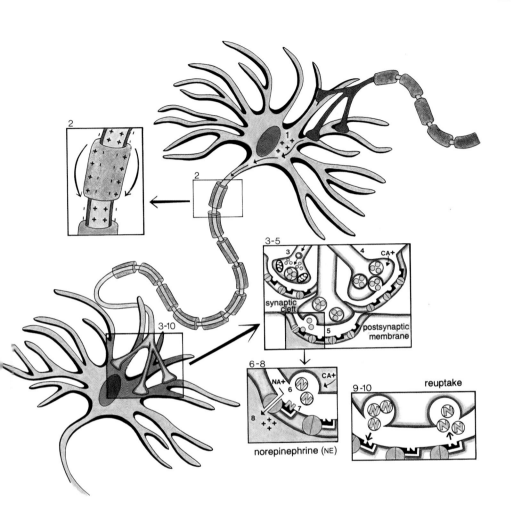

neuron. When it binds it either speeds (excites) the cell's firing rate by shortening the intervals between firing or slows (inhibits) the cell's firing rate by increasing the time between firings.

8. Okay. Neurotransmitter and receptor connect; more sodium, potassium or chloride ion channel stuff happens; the neurotransmitter does its thing—speeds up or slows down the cell firing rate—and BOOM! End transmission.

9. This is *not* a leisurely process. The neurotransmitter's gone almost before it hits the ground, and the synapse is ready for the next *INCOMING!* nerve impulse. (*See color gallery.*)

THERE ARE THEORIES about the different ways neurotransmitters might clear out of the synapse. Everyone pretty much agrees that uptake, also called reuptake, is primary. That's when neurotransmitters get sucked back into the presynaptic neuron they came from—the brain's own biogenic amine recycling program. The other theories involve any neurotransmitter molecules that miss the uptake express. They may get broken down by enzymes, or the brain's still-mysterious glial cells may suck them up in a separate process the same way ushers clear theater aisles during movie credits, or maybe they wander off into the brain.

"THERE'S THINGS GOIN' ON THAT YOU DON'T KNOW"[38]

> **"I am tired of all this thing called science... We have spent millions in that sort of thing for the last few years, and it is time it should be stopped."**—Senator Simon Cameron (PA), demanding that funding for the Smithsonian Institution be cut, 1861.[39]

A LOT OF SMART PEOPLE worked like sharecroppers for centuries so I could breeze through their research, picking out stuff I think might be interesting and useful to anyone who's ever used LSD and wondered why walls breathe

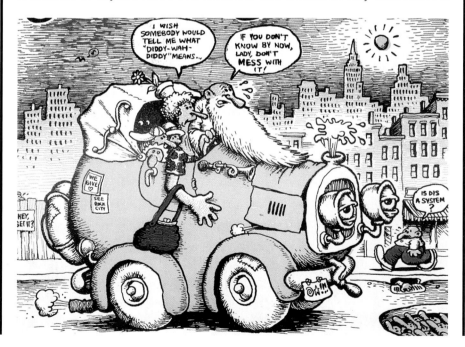

and fingers (at the very least) leave Day Glo trails in the air behind them. Or why every tiny thing that happens seems like a *very* esoteric, labyrinthine cosmic gag. That's okay. Researchers must appreciate any legitimate use of their findings, which in the science community are all more bricks in a massive wall of theory. And no one can ever *prove* a theory once and for all, then walk away from etched stone, brushing off the fine dust of truth. Even the best theories are history if enough people produce the right number of contradictory findings.

That everything's a theory is easier to believe in neuroscience and drug development than in medicine, for example, where the M.D.s so confidently deal with everything from Asian flu to open-heart surgery. But get one or two blocks south of the routine ailments and you're Linda Blair as Reagan MacNeil in *The Exorcist*,[40] shrieking through another spinal tap on your way to an exorcism with Satan and a couple of Jesuit priests in Georgetown. All that uncertainty—it's easier to see it coming if you know what to look for.

Lots of scientists hate it when some layman characterizes their life work as a theory. But the best of them know they can't be sure of anything and how to say so. One of these is Solomon Snyder, M.D., director of the Department of Neuroscience and a professor of neuroscience, pharmacology and psychiatry at Johns Hopkins University in Baltimore. He's written books like *Drugs and the Brain*, *Uses of Marijuana* and *Biological Aspects of Mental Disorder.*

THIS IS FROM <u>DRUGS AND THE BRAIN</u>:

> In this book I have tried to describe what modern neurotransmitter research is currently revealing about the actions of the principal drugs that influence the brain. I must emphasize, however, that, while the mechanisms described herein are either currently accepted theories or likely hypotheses, readers would be wrong to consider them ironclad certainties.... The mechanisms for psychoactive drug actions are as well understood as the actions of almost any other class of drugs. Again, *we do not know for certain* [his emphasis] exactly how the brain regulates specific behaviors, but we can formulate some educated guesses, and as long as they stand up to the trials we devise to test them, we can use these educated guesses as the basis for the next important advances in understanding.[41]

THAT'S WHAT YOU GET IN *Trips*—a look at how researchers *think* neurotransmitters and receptors and action potentials and ion channels work in the brain. Of all the scientists I've talked to over 10 years, particle physicists and hallucinogen researchers seem most comfortable admitting there are things they don't know, and why not? It doesn't mean they're not brilliant or they haven't worked hard.

Here's what it does mean. Admitting they don't know exactly how or where drugs work in the brain, by what mechanisms or with what long-term effects would make it impossible for any federal researchers or regulatory officials to issue edicts and make proclamations about the absolute safety or danger of *any* drug. Given the tendencies of regulatory officials to do just that, you can see how they might resist being caught uncertain in public about anything. But they still **DON'T KNOW.**

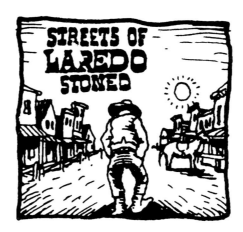

Chapter3

EARLY RESEARCHERS: PIONEERS ARE
THE ONES WITH ARROWS IN THEIR BACKS

1938-1943: ALBERT HOFMANN MEETS LSD[42]

LSD COMES FROM ERGOT, a parasitic fungus of the genus *Claviceps pur-purea* that grows on wild grasses, rye and other grain-producing plants. Fungus-infected kernels grow into light brown curved pegs that stick out of the husk. In the early Middle Ages ergot was a poison that affected many thousands of people. Order of St. Anthony members treated most patients, so people called the disease St. Anthony's Fire. Starting in the Middle Ages, midwives used ergot to speed up childbirth. In the 18th century, chemists tried to isolate and make drugs from the compounds that affected childbirth. Over time, ergot became a rich source of remedies.

In 1917, Professor Arthur Stoll founded the Sandoz company's pharmaceutical department, and ergot research became a main topic in his Basel, Switzerland-based lab. Soon he isolated an alkaloid he called *ergotamine* that had uterine and childbirth effects, but the really specific uterine

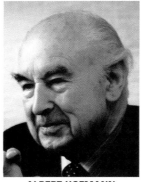

ALBERT HOFMANN

ergot alkaloid, ergobasin, wasn't isolated in labs in the United States, England and at Sandoz until 1932-1934.

About this time, Sandoz chemist Albert Hofmann finished other work and asked Stoll if he could work with ergot. His first goal was to partially synthesize ergobasin, whose chemical structure was lysergic acid propanolamide. Lysergic acid was the common nucleus of all medicinally important ergot alkaloids. Hofmann found a way to make lysergic acid amides, then linked lysergic acid with propanolamine and got a compound identical to ergobasin. It was the first time anyone synthesized a natural ergot alkaloid. A chemist who synthesized a natural product could use the same process to chemically modify the natural compound.

Hofmann synthesized lots of ergobasin analogs in 1938. These included lysergic acid butanolamide (Methergine) to treat postpartum bleeding. The 25th compound in this series of chemical modifications was lysergic acid diethylamide, a compound that seemed to stimulate blood circulation and respiration. In German it was *Lysergsäure-diäthylamid*, or LSD-25. But Sandoz top management didn't find the animal research too exciting, so they stopped testing LSD. Meanwhile, Hofmann isolated new ergot derivatives, and two became components of new Sandoz drugs.

- ● hydrogen (H)
- ○ carbon (c)
- ● oxygen (o)
- ○ nitrogen (N)
- ● phosphorus (P)
- ● chlorine (cl)
- ● fluorine (f)

LSD

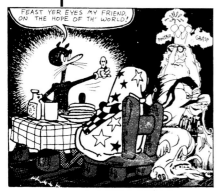

Five years went by and Hofmann couldn't forget the abandoned LSD-25. On April 16, 1943, he decided to repeat the LSD-25 synthesis, and while he was working, he abruptly entered another world. From Hofmann's book,

LSD: MY PROBLEM CHILD:

The surroundings had changed in a strange way, and had become luminous, more expres-

sive. I felt uneasy and went home, where I wanted to rest. Lying on the couch with closed eyes because I experienced daylight as unpleasantly glaring, I perceived an uninterrupted stream of fantastic pictures, with an intense kaleidoscopic play of colors. After some hours this strange but not unpleasant condition faded away. [43]

HOFMANN FIGURED SOMETHING he'd worked with in the lab caused the bizarre experience, but he couldn't understand how. Absorbed through the skin, maybe? Three days later he tried it again—just to test his assumption. It was April 19th. To purify the LSD he'd used dichloroethylene, so he tried snorting dichloroethylene fumes. Nothing. LSD was the only other candidate. He carefully mixed 250 mcg (a common '60s street dose; about twice the strength of a '90s dose) of lysergic acid diethylamide tartrate with water and drank it. Forty minutes later he was dizzy, anxious, having visual distortions, symptoms of paralysis and—an effect of LSD that doesn't get too much press—an urge to laugh. So LSD had caused whatever had happened to him a few days earlier. Only this time it was more intense. He asked his lab assistant to help him get home. And no wonder.

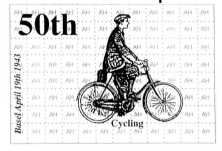

Source: Dr. Malcolm Lader, Institute of Psychiatry, De Crespigny Park, Denmark Hill, London. Used with permission.

Hofmann lived four miles away and had to ride a bicycle. So they climbed on the bikes and Hofmann did four miles coming on to the world's first dose of synthetic LSD. As a tribute in 1993, a handful of Brits printed sheets of blotter acid to commemorate the 50 years since Hofmann's wild ride home.

LATER, HOFMANN DESCRIBED HIS EXPERIENCE IN A BOOK, *LSD: MY PROBLEM CHILD*:

Everything in my field of vision wavered and was distorted as if seen in a curved mirror. I had lost the feeling of time which resulted in the sensation of being unable to move from the spot, although my assistant said we traveled very rapidly. At home I asked my companion to summon our family doctor and request milk from our neighbor. In spite of my delirious condition, I was still capable of clear and effective thinking—milk is a nonspecific antidote for poisoning... Everything in the room spun around and familiar objects and the furniture assumed grotesque, threatening forms. They were in continuous motion, animated, as if driven by an inner restlessness... When the neighbor brought milk, she was no longer Mrs. Meyer but a malevolent witch with a colored mask.

The substance with which I had wanted to experiment had become a demon who vanquished me and scornfully triumphed over my will. I was seized by the dreadful fear of having become insane... By the time the doctor arrived, the climax of my despondent condition had already passed... He could not detect any abnormal symptoms other than extremely dilated pupils. Pulse, blood pressure and breathing were all normal...

Slowly I came back from a weird, strange world to reassuring everyday reality. The horror softened and gave way to a feeling of good fortune and gratitude. Now...I could begin to enjoy the unprecedented colors and plays of shapes that persisted behind my closed eye....I then slept, to awake the next morning refreshed and with a clear head, though still somewhat physically tired. When I later walked out into the garden, in which the sun shone after a spring rain, everything glistened and sparkled in an enchanting new light. The world seemed as if newly created.[44]

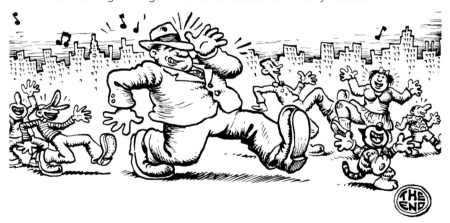

THREE MORE SANDOZ SCIENTISTS took LSD at a third of Hofmann's dose because no one had ever heard of a psychoactive compound that produced effects at such a low dose. LSD made them believers. "After the discovery of the effects on human psyche," Hofmann said, "one could expect that such a substance would receive an important place in brain research."

This segment comes mainly from *OSS: The Secret History of America's First Central Intelligence Agency* by R. Harris Smith.

HOFMANN WASN'T WRONG. But one of the weirdest places LSD ended up was in the research labs of the Office of Strategic Services—OSS. America's first central intelligence agency was led by its 58-year-old founder, William 'Wild Bill' Donovan, a millionaire Wall Street lawyer. OSS was born six months after Japan attacked Pearl Harbor. About three seconds later, America was emotionally, economically and politically hip-deep in the military crisis of World

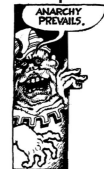

War II, and someone was thinking that Wild Bill Donovan—also a World War I hero who held the country's three highest military decorations—was just the guy to head OSS.

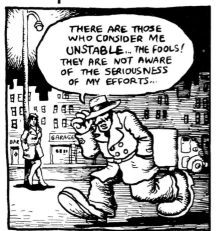

Some people say Donovan ran OSS "like a country editor," but the war begged for fresh thinking and not what you'd call organizational hierarchy to stand in the way.[46] One in four of OSS's 9,000 military personnel were commissioned officers, most of them junior. As long as everyone did their work, no one bothered with military regs.

There was no saluting and they wore whatever they wanted to. They grew long hair and beards, or sprouted long mustaches and shaved their heads. Insubordination was a way of life. Standard operating procedures were taboo. Donovan was famous for his willingness to listen to any "eccentric schemer with a plan for secret operations—from phosphorescent foxes to incendiary bats." Some of it even worked. But the line is always thin between unstructured thinking and instability.[47]

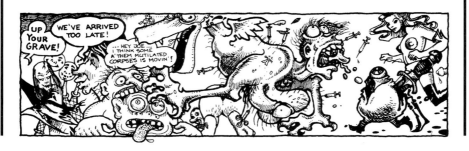

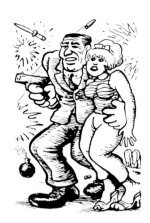

"The whole nature of [OSS] functions was particularly inviting to psychopathic characters," said Donovan's former psychological chief. "It involved sensation, intrigue, the idea of being a mysterious man with secret knowledge."[48]

In 1942, Donovan asked a handful of top U.S. scientists to work on a high-level secret project to develop a truth serum for intelligence interrogations.[49] He wanted to be able to "break down the psychological defenses of enemy spies and POWs" so they'd spill their guts and disclose classified information. The scientists started with a potent extract of marijuana and went on to stronger drugs. It wasn't long before their search for a truth serum started looking just like a search for the ultimate mind-control drug.[50]

After the war OSS sort of evolved into the new Central Intelligence Agency (CIA). But the place felt a lot like OSS. The CIA Office of Policy Coordination handled political subversion. The CIA Office of Special Operations handled espionage and collected intelligence. That, in the early 1950s, was where LSD came in.[51]

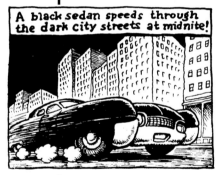

Meanwhile, in 1948, the OSS/CIA guys were gearing up for all the creepy stuff they were going to try in the 1950s and '60s—more drug testing, this time on unwitting CIA employees, military officers *and* U.S. citizens. They explored sensory deprivation, sleep teaching and ESP; subliminal projection and electronic brain stimulation; and brain effects of magnetic fields, ultrasonic vibrations and other radiant energy. The same year a research team at the Cleveland Clinic in Ohio discovered something that eventually would be critical to hallucinogen research.[52]

 MORE ABOUT SEROTONIN: IT'S 5-HT

IRVINE PAGE, research division director at the Cleveland Clinic, led the team that isolated from blood serum an endogenous chemical they called serotonin. Scientists had known for 100 years that some substance was in there causing smooth-muscle organs to contract, but no one had been able to get

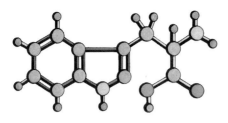

TRYPTOPHAN

a handle on it. When Page's team first isolated serotonin, they thought it might cause high blood pressure. Later they identified serotonin in the central nervous system.

In 1949 the team concluded that serotonin's active ingredient was 5-hydroxytryptamine (5-HT). This was synthesized in 1951 and had all the properties of natural serotonin. By now everyone knew serotonin was in lots of different cells, and only 1 or 2 percent of the body's supply was in the brain. But 5-HT couldn't cross the blood-brain barrier—the brain's own electrochemical security gate—so they realized brain cells must make their own serotonin. To do that the cells needed an amino acid called tryptophan, the basis of serotonin synthesis. The body gets tryptophan mainly from the diet, so missing out on dietary tryptophan can lower brain serotonin levels big time. Serotonin metabolism goes like this: tryptophan enters the body, then in the right cells starts getting chemically oxidized to 5-hydroxytryptophan (5-HTP), then 5-hydroxytryptamine (serotonin) then to serotonin's breakdown product, 5-hydroxyindoleacetic acid (5-HIAA).

WHEN PAGE'S TEAM also found serotonin in the central nervous system, a theory bobbed to the surface—that some forms of mental illness might come from biochemical screw-ups that happen while the body's making its own serotonin. The theory started looking pretty good when researchers realized that

◎ A tranquilizing compound, reserpine, reduced serotonin in the brain

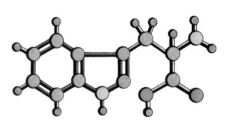

TRYPTOPHAN

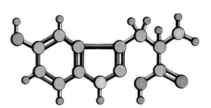

5-HYDROXTRYPTAMINE (5-HTP)

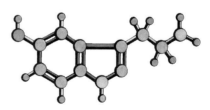

SEROTONIN

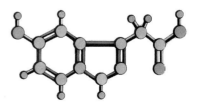

5-HYDROXYINDOLEACETIC ACID (5-HIAA)

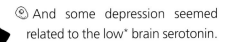

 And some depression seemed related to the low* brain serotonin.

Although a theory is not confirmed fact, some of these theories still make sense, and there's lots more evidence to support them.[53]

The histories of serotonin and LSD have intertwined ever since.[54]

LSD HIT THE UNITED STATES IN 1949, and the scientific community loved it. In less than a decade LSD had major credibility among psychiatrists, and it was no passing fad. Over the next few years, LSD therapists wrote more than 1,000 clinical papers discussing 40,000 patients. They got good results when they used LSD to treat really resistant psychiatric conditions like frigidity and other sexual aberrations. Some saw dramatically decreased autistic symptoms in withdrawn children who got LSD therapy. Others found that LSD

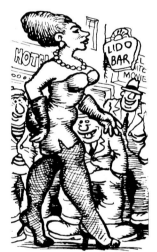

eased physical and psychological distress for terminal cancer patients, and helped them deal with their impending deaths. Even some chronic alcoholics did well after high-dose LSD therapy. The improvement rate for some was higher with LSD therapy than with traditional methods, and its risks were more appealing than the ones that came with

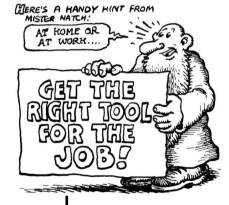

electroshock, lobotomy (ow), and antipsychotic drugs.

---

*Scientists talk about 'levels' of serotonin and other neurotransmitters being high or low, or about a drug that 'raises' or 'lowers' neurotransmitter levels. What they're really talking about are levels of *activity* (how many times a cell fires per second or nanosecond) in neural pathways that use serotonin as a neurotransmitter, not the absolute amount of serotonin in the brain. From Kramer, author's note, *Listening to Prozac*: 326.

PART II

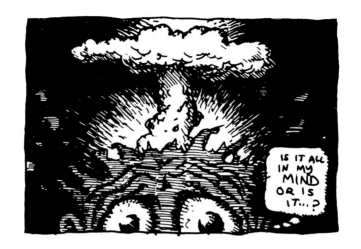

Chapter 4

THE 1950s: HALLUCINOGENS— AS CLOSE AS YOU GET TO PSYCHOSIS WITHOUT BEING PSYCHO YOURSELF

NOW LSD PSYCHOTHERAPY STARTED getting interesting. The CIA secret research guys thought so too. With help from the Army's secret research guys, CIA escalated its no-holds-barred search for the ultimate truth drug, shoes crunching through the smoking debris of the U.S. government's new code of medical ethics—that researchers shouldn't use people as subjects without their full consent—burned beyond recognition. But as a group, federal neuropharmacologists seemed cosmically unequipped to *get* the nature of LSD.

Then there was DMT—another gift from the African rain forest to The Streets by way of the Congo, South America, Budapest, Milan, Washington and San Francisco.

 LSD, PSYCHOTHERAPY & ALCOHOLISM

It was 1950 and LSD had been in the United States for a year when the general perception of it as a psychotomimetic—a drug that mimics psychosis—

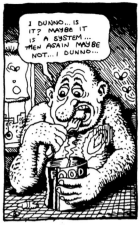

started to change. The first hint[55] was when researchers A.K. Busch and W.C. Johnson published an article in *Diseases of the Nervous System* suggesting LSD might help patients in psychotherapy, but not because it mimicked psychosis. They'd noticed that actual psychotic patients in delirium could sometimes verbalize repressed conflicts, so they decided to investigate new drugs that might cause temporary delirium. Sandoz offered LSD, and Busch and Johnson studied it in patients. After a preliminary investigation, they said LSD might help chronically withdrawn patients and shorten the course of psychotherapy for others.

In 1953, German psychiatrist Walter Frederking published one of the first European articles on LSD as part of psychotherapy. In what came to be known as *psycholytic* (from the Greek words for 'mind' and 'to loosen') therapy, he used low doses of LSD to shorten therapy, ease mood problems or memory blocks and get patients to something called catharsis—a way to relieve anxiety and tension by bringing repressed memories and emotions to consciousness. Over the next few years, psychiatrists around the world who used LSD in therapy report-

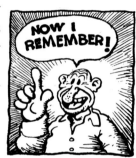

ed similar results. Soon a group of European psychiatrists formed an association of psycholytic therapists—who used low-to-moderate doses of LSD over two to 100 sessions to shorten and improve psychoanalysis and psychoanalytic therapy.

Psycholytic therapy grew in Europe and the United States and, from 1953 to 1967, research papers documented good results. But most therapists still saw LSD as a kind of toxin. Even those who reported good results started work assuming LSD would create toxic delirium in patients.

Not that the usual therapy-accelerators were much better. Some side effects of treatments like amobarbital (a long-acting tranquilizer), sodium pentothal, insulin shock and electroshock (ow) could turn patients into extras for the graveyard scene in *Night of the Living Dead*. But LSD patients remembered everything that happened in therapy, which was critical to integrating their new insights into everyday consciousness.

As early as the '50s, a few researchers noticed that LSD wasn't just a psychotomimetic; they started promoting a more radical view and used it to develop LSD therapies for untreatable disorders like schizophrenia and alcoholism. One group included Abram Hoffer, M.D., Ph.D., British psychiatrist Humphrey Osmond, and a small group of researchers in Saskatchewan, Canada.[56] Hoffer and Osmond were pioneers of North American research on hallucinogens, and are regular characters in time-lines and chronicles that deal with the evolution of psychedelics.

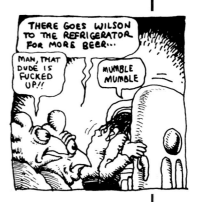

ABRAM HOFFER SEZ

From a November 1995 interview with Abram Hoffer, 80, at his office in Victoria, British Columbia, where he practices macro-molecular medicine.

"[Humphrey] Osmond brought across from England the idea that LSD might mimic schizophrenia. In [World War II] Osmond was a Navy physician. After the war he... took psychiatric training. Then he met a colleague, John Smythies, who told him that some asthmatics who inhaled adrenaline for asthma became psychotic. So they got interested in mescaline research.

"Now Osmond and Smythies thought there might be something in the body [endogenous] that has the psychiatric properties of mescaline. They wanted to investigate that question [but the medical establishment] laughed at them, thought it was crazy. So Osmond and Smythies left England and came to Saskatchewan. [In Canada,] Osmond presented the idea to me and, since I knew nothing about psychiatry, it seemed like a pretty nice idea. He and I began to work on it together.

"We got interested in the hallucinogens. There were very few then—mescaline was one, and LSD was becoming popular. If I gave you 500 milligrams of mescaline, you probably wouldn't enjoy the next 24 hours—too long. LSD is more controllable. You usually get off within an hour and you're out in seven or eight hours. We felt it would be easier to work with, so we turned to LSD.

"At the time [Osmond and I] were investigating schizophrenia, and [LSD-induced] psychosis was as close as we could get to it without becoming psychotic ourselves. We began to study normal subjects with LSD and took it ourselves. It's all written up in The Hallucinogens.[57] I only took LSD twice, but not to have a transcendental experience. We wanted to know what it was like to be schizophrenic. How can you talk to a patient if you don't understand what he's going through?

Then one night in 1950 or '51, after a cold, noisy flight to Ottawa with Osmond, Hoffer got an idea about using LSD to treat alcoholics.

"I couldn't sleep and when I can't sleep, I think. I was thinking about LSD and suddenly it occurred to me—What if we could make an alcoholic have a controlled delirium tremens?

"It's said an alcoholic has to 'hit bottom' [emotionally, physically, economically, socially or spiritually] before he changes. That's dangerous because hitting bottom, you tend to...die. But what if we could make him have the hitting-bottom experience without dying? Second, when you have delirium tremens and come out of it, you often remember snatches of it but you don't remember the whole thing. It's like a bad dream—it fades away. We didn't like that either. Then we said, Let's try LSD. Let's see if we can make them have such a horrible experience under LSD that we can tell them later on, 'If you keep drinking, that's going to happen again.' Let's frighten them. That was the idea.

"I discussed it with my colleague and we both thought it was worth trying. We began to treat alcoholics with LSD, trying to make them have this absolutely horrible experience. To our amazement we found that we couldn't. In spite of everything we tried, they'd have a good experience, a psychedelic experience. They enjoyed it, they felt good, they saw strange things, they were excited about it. Osmond said, We'll have to give it a different name. It's not what we want but we can't deny the facts; this is what's happening. And he coined the word 'psychedelic' [mind manifesting]. We'd been using the psychiatric medical approach and that was...the stick. We said, Let's use the carrot, the psychedelic approach—see if we can make every alcoholic have a really good transcendental experience.

"Then we introduced things like a nice room, pictures, nice music, kind nurses, kind doctors who would be sympathetic and who could control and support the patient. To our delight this worked even better. We began to see results. I'll give you a classic example of an alcoholic...a man who never responded to treatment no matter what we did. He didn't get better but was always an agreeable guy—Yes doc. Sure doc. Tell me what to do and I'll do it. Except he'd never stop drinking and was in and out of hospitals. I went to him. John, how about trying LSD? He said, Sure doc, anything. John had a superior image of himself; he knew he had a superior brain. LSD wasn't going to touch him so he didn't mind doing it just to please us. We gave him 200 micrograms and nothing happened.

"A week later he agreed to try it again. I said, We're going to give you more, is that okay? He said, Okay doc. We gave him 400 micrograms [ow]* at 9 a.m. and by 10 a.m. it should have been working. He was suddenly very tense and couldn't talk. We watched him but nothing seemed to happen. The next morning he said that around 11 a.m. God had come to him and said, John, no more. He never touched

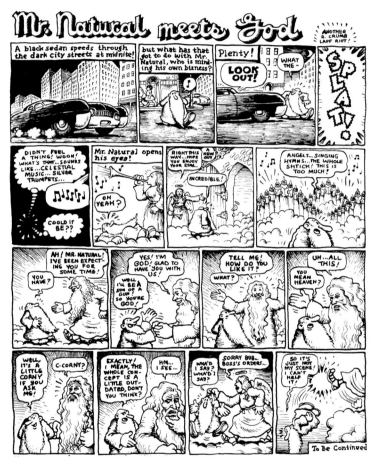

alcohol after that. In fact, he became a minister. It was a striking case—what you call transcendental."

"We always used LSD therapy as an introduction to AA. We said, 'After you have this experience you've got to go to AA.' By this time we were close friends of Bill W.

---

*Regular street doses are like this: 75-125 mcg from the mid-1970s to the 1990s; 250-350 mcg in the 1960s.

[cofounder with Dr. Bob Smith of Alcoholics Anonymous (AA) in 1935] so I knew all about AA… After we began to see what was happening with the alcoholics, we studied [the nature of the spiritual or transcendental experience] that changed their minds about drinking. Bill learned about LSD from us."

While the work with alcoholics continued, Hoffer discovered some-

INDOLES

An indole—sometimes called an indole nucleus—is the chemical basis of lots of biologically active substances like serotonin and tryptophan. It's a building block of tryptamines because adding a short carbon chain to the indole nucleus creates a tryptamine. By 1972, researchers knew about more than 500 naturally occurring indole alkaloids. By 1980 there were 1,200. By 1995, lots more pharmacologically and structurally diverse compounds were on the list, which included tryptophan, an essential amino acid; serotonin, a neurotransmitter; and the hallucinogens ibogaine, LSD, DMT and psilocybin.[58]

THREE TAKES ON LSD PSYCHOTHERAPY[59]

PSYCHOTOMIMETIC (PSYCHOSIS MIMICKING) THERAPY

Because LSD was discovered in a drug lab instead of a rain forest, researchers used scientific methods to quantify and characterize its effects. LSD had such a huge effect on mental function that researchers said it induced toxic psychosis. Pretty soon, people who didn't know much else about LSD thought they knew that its effects mimicked psychosis. Patients took LSD in white-tiled, fluorescently lit, sterile clinics and hospitals. They had no music; cold, shiny tubes and wires clung to their bodies and they had to sit or lie on hospital beds. The doctors wore white coats.

PSYCHOLYTIC (MIND LOOSENING) THERAPY

Psycholytic therapists use LSD and other hallucinogens in low-to-moderate doses (30 to 200 mcg) to shorten and speed up psychoanalysis and psychoanalytical therapy. It involves 2 to 100 drug sessions while the patient's in therapy.

PSYCHEDELIC (MIND MANIFESTING) THERAPY

Psychedelic therapists use high doses of LSD to encourage dramatic, overwhelming changes in consciousness that lead to peak experiences and new levels of awareness. The physical environment [setting] is comfortable, aesthetically pleasing and has great music.

thing about LSD that started federal research dollars flowing: "Now I was a biochemist and we have a well-known rule in chemistry that compounds with similar structures tend to have similar properties. We said, Is it possible?... Osmond said, *Maybe there's something in common with all these.*"

"I wrote down their chemical structure and to my amazement—and I remember distinctly to this day, sitting in our home, a very small house, my wife and two small kids—I'm working at the kitchen table and suddenly get this flash. There's something common to these. I said, *My God, the indole structure is common to them all.* Indoles were known to be present in the body; [the essential amino acid] tryptophan's an indole. So we had our first meeting and got our first grant.

"We got $23,000 in 1951 from the federal government and started our research. Between 1954 and 1960 we took LSD and gave it to thousands of subjects. We were the largest group in Canada working with LSD. We treated 2,000 alcoholics, experimenting with the best dose. For normal people it's 100 micrograms, for alcoholics it's 200-400 mcg.

"We experimented with various doses but never went high enough to cause confusion. And since we didn't want to harm any of our patients, we had a firm rule: if someone ever had schizophrenia or a first-order relative who was schizophrenic, we'd never give them LSD because they're the ones who had bad trips. Of the thousands of people we gave LSD to, we didn't damage a single person. Even today, on occasion, a patient will come in and say, I had LSD from you in 1960 and I haven't been drinking since."

◢ CIA, DOD, LSD
YOU CAN'T HANDLE THE TRUTH [DRUG]

> This segment comes mainly from *Acid Dreams: The CIA, LSD and the Sixties Rebellion* by Martin Lee and Bruce Shlain (Grove Press, 1985). I've never read a better book on the subject.

> **"We must always remember to thank the CIA and the Army for LSD. That's what people forget... They [studied and used] LSD to control people and what they did was give us freedom. Sometimes it works in mysterious ways its wonders to perform."**—John Lennon, 1980[60]

AFTER WORLD WAR II, the CIA picked up where OSS left off. It was 1951 and PROJECT BLUEBIRD was the first major drug-testing program. Later that year it became OPERATION ARTICHOKE—same game, different name. CIA researchers still wanted a perfect "speech-inducing substance."[61]

In the early 1950s, the CIA was still green and growing. Its operating philosophy, inherited from OSS, inspired a Beavis-and-Butthead-like attitude among the mind-control researchers, who really wanted to deliver that truth drug. The CIA sent people to places so primitive they didn't have McDonald's franchises just to fetch rare herbs and botanicals. Over time they studied a

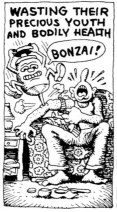
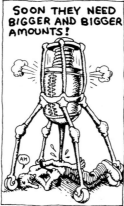
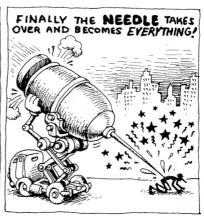

"veritable pharmacopoeia of drugs"[62] to see what cocaine, morphine, ether, benzedrine, mescaline, heroin, (beverage) alcohol, and the roasting-on-a-spit-in-hell pain of withdrawal from heroin and other addictive drugs would do to people with secrets.[63] Then they discovered LSD.

Working under PROJECT ARTICHOKE, a CIA psychiatrist suggested LSD might be just the thing for interrogating the enemy. What the hell—they'd tried everything else. CIA researchers dosed 12 unwitting subjects with 100-150 micrograms (mcg) and tested them in mock interrogations. It seemed to work.

For a while they thought LSD was their truth drug, but research continued and they realized it wasn't exactly a classic truth serum. They couldn't get good information from people on LSD because it tended

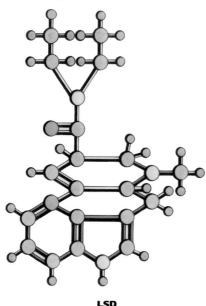

LSD

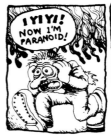
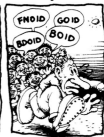

to cause "marked anxiety and loss of reality contact." For the clueless subjects, time, place and body image were totally distorted, and they often ended up with "full-blown paranoid reactions."[64]

More bad news. An enemy agent who realized he'd been drugged might stop talking completely. And—though LSD gave subjects more anxiety

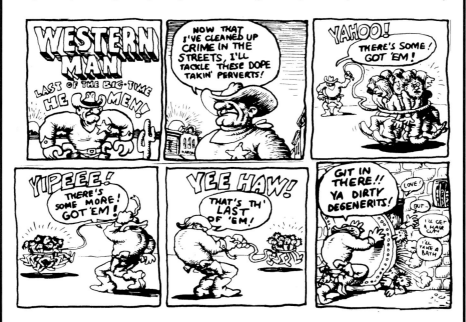

than anything else—some had "delusions of grandeur and omnipotence. An entire operation might backfire if someone had an ecstatic or transcendental experience and became convinced that he could defy his interrogators indefinitely."[65]

The ARTICHOKE guys were so afraid the Soviets and Red Chinese would stumble on psychedelic interrogation that they kept using LSD even though they knew it didn't work. But they did try new approaches, including one that security officers suggested—using LSD as a sort of vaccine against interrogation. If they couldn't trust information that came from research subjects on LSD, their own operatives, if captured by enemies, might use LSD to keep from spilling their own guts in enemy interrogations. Then one day the ARTICHOKE guys realized the enemy could use LSD "to produce anxiety or terror in medically unsophisticated subjects" who couldn't tell LSD "from actual insanity."

Soon LSD trips were a regular part of training, to give some operatives experience with hallucinogen effects on themselves and co-workers. It didn't take security officials long to propose LSD screening for all CIA trainee-volunteers, and the CIA medical office wanted every CIA employee to take the test. In 1953 the ARTICHOKE committee verbally agreed. Over the next few years lots of CIA operatives tried LSD, some more than once.[66] CIA documents said the agency used LSD during interrogations from the mid-1950s through the early 1960s.[67] Every now and then, the CIA got help with its drug-testing programs from the former Federal Narcotics Bureau and the Food and Drug Administration.

When the CIA first got interested in LSD, only a handful of U.S. scientists were researching hallucinogens. But the market for LSD research grants boomed as money[68] started spurting through CIA conduits. By the mid-1950s lots of independent investigators were studying LSD and other hallucinogens, and all were monitored by CIA field offices.[69]

IT'S NOT A JOB, IT'S A PSYCHOTIC EPISODE[70]

Around the same time, Army, Navy and Air Force military intelligence types heard about LSD. By the mid-1950s all the services were funding LSD studies. The Army's Chemical Warfare Service at Edgewood Arsenal stockpiled

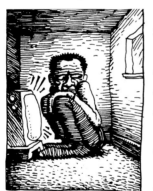
big supplies of LSD and other drugs, and synthesized hallucinogens the outside world still might not know about. Army spokesmen went public about using LSD on a large scale against wartime adversaries, and showed members of Congress and the press a film of soldiers who couldn't march in a straight line after having their morning coffee with cream and (surprise!) LSD.

The Army liked to call it the *humane* way to defeat enemies, even while they were setting up covert field operations overseas and creating their own victims. Like 22-year-old James Thornwell, a black American soldier stationed in France in 1961. He was assigned to an LSD interrogation project and torture fest called OPERATION THIRD CHANCE after being suspected of stealing classified documents. First, Thornwell and others got six weeks of what the Army called *extreme stress*—beatings; solitary confinement; no food, water or bathrooms; and continuous verbal abuse. Then Thornwell got a surprise dose of LSD. While he was tripping, his interrogators threatened "to extend [his fragmented] state indefinitely," according to an internal Army document, "even to a permanent condition of insanity."[71]

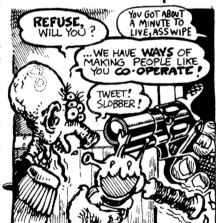

CIA & PRISONERS OF [THE COLD, COLD] WAR

Meanwhile, four years into MK-ULTRA (formerly OPERATION ARTICHOKE) and 20 more to go, the U.S. formally adopted a code of military ethics based on the 1947 Nuremberg Code—the statement of medical ethics that evolved after World War II from the Nazi war crime trials in Germany. The military code of ethics said clearly that medical research should be conducted only with subjects' full consent and knowledge.[72]

1952-1963: LSD TESTS ON PRISONERS. With money channeled through the Office of Naval Research, researchers tested LSD and similar drugs on prisoners at the U.S. Public Health Service Hospital in Lexington, Kentucky. They wanted a substitute for the painkiller codeine, even though LSD had no painkilling properties. Research coordinator Dr. Harris Isbell secretly stayed in touch with the CIA and arranged their overseas drug buys from European manufacturers who thought they were shipping to U.S. public health officials.[73]

1953: FRANK OLSON, LSD & THE CIA. In November 1953 a group of CIA and Army technicians gathered for a three-day work retreat at a remote hunting lodge near Fort Detrick, Maryland. On the second day, MK-ULTRA program director Sidney Gottlieb dosed after-dinner cocktails with LSD. As the drug started working, Gottlieb announced that he'd spiked their drinks and they'd better hang on. By that time most of the guys were screaming with laughter or looking at their hands and couldn't hold coherent conversations. Frank Olson, an Army biochemist whose work involved biological warfare research, was part of the group. He was usually friendly and a family man but he went home quiet and withdrawn. After the retreat he slid into a deep depression. At work he asked his boss to fire him for messing up the experiment at the retreat. Olson's superiors called the CIA and the agency sent him to New York to see Dr. Harold Abramson, a physician, Columbia University professor, one of the CIA's top LSD researchers, and a part-time Army Chemical Corps consultant.

But Olson needed a real psychiatrist. For a few weeks he told Abramson his fears—the CIA drugged his coffee to keep him awake at night, people plotted against him and he heard voices at all hours commanding him to throw away his wallet. Abramson reported that Olson was "mired in a psychotic state... with delusions of persecution" that the LSD experience had

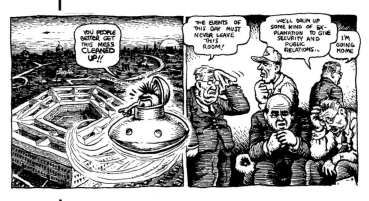

crystallized. The CIA arranged to move Olson to Chestnut Lodge, a sanitarium in Rockville, Maryland, with hot and cold running CIA-cleared psychiatrists.

On his last night in New York, Olson checked into a room at the Statler Hilton with a CIA agent who'd been assigned to watch him. Sometime before dawn, Olson plunged through a closed window to the sidewalk 10 floors down. The CIA elaborately covered up the details of what they called his suicide. CIA director Allen Dulles briefly suspended the in-house LSD testing program, ran an internal investigation, then gently reprimanded Gottlieb and his team for using bad judgment and kept it out of their personnel files.[74] In 1977, Olson's family was invited to the White House for a formal apology, and Congress passed a bill to pay Mrs. Olson and her three children $750,000 in compensation.*,[75]

1955: PRISONER EXPERIMENTS WITH LSD. In 1955, Gottlieb asked pharmacologist Carl Pfeiffer to give LSD to prisoners at the federal penitentiary in Atlanta and at New Jersey's Bordentown Reformatory. Pfeiffer accepted $25,000 a year through the Geschikter Foundation for Medical Research, a CIA front. For 11 years he gave LSD to 80 or 100 prisoners and, in a 1977 interview, Pfeiffer would say he had prisoner consent but that he didn't believe consent was always needed in "wartime conditions."[76]

1957: EXPERIMENTS ON 'CRIMINAL SEXUAL PSYCHOPATHS.' More than 140 research subjects from Detroit's Recorders Court psychiatric clinic were given LSD in 1957 to see if it made them confess hidden thoughts. The CIA chose them because criminally insane sexual psychopaths had the "kind of

---

*The Olson investigation was revisited in 1994, when Georgetown University law professor/forensic scientist James Storrs and a team from Engineering Animation Inc. (EAI) used computer animation to recreate the details of Frank Olson's death. Check it out on the Internet at http://www.eai.com.

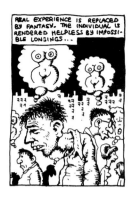

REAL EXPERIENCE IS REPLACED BY FANTASY. THE INDIVIDUAL IS RENDERED HELPLESS BY IMPOSSIBLE LONGINGS...

motivation for withholding certain information that is comparable to operational interrogative situations in the field." There was no record of prisoner consent, and doctors used tape recorders and lie detectors to question drugged prisoners. The clinic psychiatric associate doubled as CIA project manager and contacted the agency using double envelopes and a fake name. The Society for the Investigation of Human Ecology, a CIA front, funded the project.[77]

1958: SENSORY DEPRIVATION & DRUG RESEARCH. The Allain Memorial Institute at McGill University in Canada used CIA funds to do bizarre sleep experiments on schizophrenics. Without their consent, Dr. Ewen Cameron knocked patients out for a week at a time and gave them electroshock therapy and LSD to erase old behavior patterns. Nine of 10 patients eventually sued the government.[78]

 SEROTONIN: NOW WE'RE GETTING SOMEWHERE

Meanwhile, in the brain research arena, in the mid-1950s, two scientists finally found a way to map serotonin neurons. They published their work in 1965. Now other serotonin researchers could see what they were doing and it made a difference. As mapping techniques improved, researchers could see that most serotonin neuron cell bodies lay in clusters in or near the midline or raphe regions of the pons and upper brainstem.

upper
brain stem

pons

midline raphe region

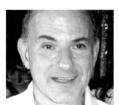 **SEROTONIN & HALLUCINOGENS**

"When I learned about the discovery of mapping the serotonergic neurons," said Aghajanian, "I thought a possible interpretation of the biochemical effects—which amounted to a decreased turnover of serotonin—could be that LSD causes the

GEORGE AGHAJANIAN

decreased turnover by decreasing [nerve] impulse flow. I did the first electrophysiological experiment I'd ever done in my life, just to test that hypothesis. The first time I tried it, LSD inhibited the firing of serotonergic neurons. I said, *Well, this is easy. On to the next question!*

THE GUY TALKING IS GEORGE AGHAJANIAN, an electrophysiologist and neuropharmacologist in the Departments of Psychiatry and Pharmacology, Yale University School of Medicine. It's November 1995 and he's the after-dinner speaker at a social meeting of researchers who belong to the Serotonin Club. Over clinking silverware he gives highlights from the research history of serotonin, and gets in a few good gags.

Aghajanian has spent most of his career studying psychedelics directly in animal brains, electrophysiologically. That means he uses microelectrodes to record the firing rate of individual neurons, then compares and analyzes the results.

"From the very beginning there were some simple, direct questions about how serotonin and LSD fit together, and how LSD and the other class of hallucinogens, represented by mescaline, fit together. LSD and serotonin were pretty obvious; they both had the indole nucleus. With mescaline the similarity was less obvious.

"On a research level, the questions were, and in a way still are: Does LSD have major hallucinogenic actions through an interaction with serotonin receptors? Do the two classes of hallucinogens have a common site of action? The possibilities were that the two classes of drugs could act at different sites or they could act at the same site, but the end result was the same. LSD and other indoleamine hallucinogens have potent, direct inhibitory effects on [they slow down the firing rate of] serotonin neurons in the raphe nucleus. Some researchers had already found that serotonin levels in the brain rise after LSD is present; this helps explain why.

"Then we found that mescaline and other phenethylamine hallucinogens didn't do the same thing. This was kind of bad news because it meant we had to have the more complicated hypothesis—that LSD and mescaline-type hallucinogens wouldn't have a common site of action. But the news got worse. We kept finding other kinds of drugs that did this, too, but they were clearly not hallucinogens—now we know they're 5-HT$_1$ agonists. So this was absolutely wrong as a mechanism for at least the hallucinogenic action of LSD."

AGONISTS, ANTAGONISTS & RECEPTORS

This information comes from *Drugs and the Brain* by Solomon Snyder, M.D.

AGONIST: The word comes from a Greek word that means 'to contend, to act.' An agonist acts at a receptor to make a change in the body. Morphine's an example of an opiate agonist. The change it makes is to stop pain and create a feeling of well-being.

ANTAGONIST: Chemically, an antagonist might look a lot like the agonist, but it has an opposite effect. It blocks agonist activity. So opiate antagonists like naloxone reverse the effects of opiates.

RECEPTORS: Most people talk about neurotransmission in terms of receptors, but pharmacologists call them 'receptor complexes' because to them a receptor has two parts—a binding site and a second messenger system. Brain cells communicate when neurotransmitters like serotonin are released from presynaptic neurons, cross the synaptic gap between brain cells, and bind to their receptors on postsynaptic neurons. The process sounds slow, but a neurotransmitter blasts across at 200 miles an hour, BOOM!, hits the receptor, and is gone before the next burst hits. The second messenger system goes to work when neurotransmitter and receptor bind. Its job is to relay the neurotransmitter's message—to translate that binding event into changes (like slowing down or speeding up) in the brain cell's firing rate and metabolism.

Some psychoactive drugs affect neurotransmission at the receptors. Chemically, a drug that looks enough like a neurotransmitter can bind to its receptor and mimic neurotransmitter effects. Drugs that do this are usually agonists. Antagonists are drugs that bind to a receptor and just sit there with no message, blocking neurotransmitter effects by denying them access to the receptor. And no chemical works in the brain unless it can bind to a receptor.

HOW IT WORKS: Here's how the agonist-antagonist thing works in the real world. Someone ODs on heroin—goes into a deep coma. Panic. Phone call. Ambulance. Doctors crash into the emergency room with the patient on a rolling litter. Wouldn't it be handy to have an opiate antagonist that could block heroin receptors and make it stop working in his brain? There is one— naloxone. A doctor shoots some into the patient's vein and within 30 seconds the heroin effects are reversed. The patient sits up. He's alert and back to norm...the way he was before he overdosed. It can take up to 30 minutes for some LSD antagonists to work because LSD binds so tightly that it takes time to 'pry' the LSD molecules off the $5\text{-}HT_{2A}$ receptor.

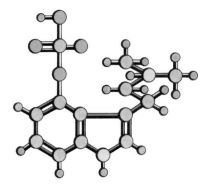

PSILOCYBIN

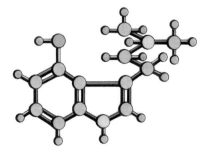

PSILOCIN

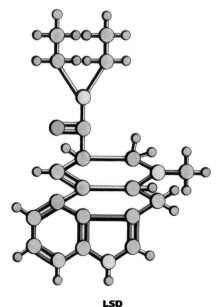

LSD

In the early 1950s, Americans R. Gordon Wasson and his wife V.P. Wasson discovered an ancient psychedelic mushroom cult in Mexico's Southern mountains. They're ethnologists, so they study cultural origins, heritage and socioeconomic systems in primitive societies. Later, in Paris, mycologist Roger Heim identified the mushrooms botanically but had a hell of a time finding a lab that could isolate their active elements. Finally, in 1957, Heim sent them to someone he knew could do it.

According to Albert Hofmann, "[Heim] hoped that in the laboratory where LSD had been discovered, the special skill would exist for a successful chemical analysis. He was right."[79] It didn't take Hofmann and co-workers long to isolate, identify and synthesize psychoactive elements from *teonanacatl*, the Mazatec Indians' magic *Psilocybe* mushroom. Hofmann's team called the compounds *psilocybin* and *psilocin* after the mushroom *Psilocybe mexicana*.

Meanwhile, Hofmann was *into* hallucinogens. In 1959, from a fellow researcher he received a package of seeds from a plant then called *Rivea corymbosa*, the sacred Aztec *ololiuqui*, a Mexican morning glory. In 1960, Hofmann identified, isolated and analyzed the active elements. They were ergot alkaloids—*lysergic acid* alkaloids.

"When we analyzed these seeds our findings seemed impossible," Hofmann said. "The psychoactive [elements] of *ololiuqui* were lysergic acid amide and lysergic acid hydroxyethylamide—nearly identical with... LSD."[80]

Until then, Hofmann and everyone else thought LSD was just synthetic—a hybrid product of laboratory chemistry. But lysergic acid alkaloids in the Mexican morning glory showed for the first time that a molecule really similar to LSD occurred naturally in a higher plant species. For Hofmann the finding was unexpected but fascinating because lysergic acid alkaloids had, until then, only been found in lower fungi in the genus *Claviceps*. Now here they were, growing wild in a higher plant species, the family *Convolvulaceae*.[81] Maybe he'd eventually find them in humans.

 ## N,N-DIMETHYLTRYPTAMINE (DMT)

DMT is the active ingredient in several hallucinogenic snuff powders, including one called *cohoba* that some South American Indians use to induce religious ecstasy. And it's a component of *ayahuasca* (vine of the soul), a hallucinogenic tea made from the *Banistereopsis caapi* vine and the *Psychotria viridis* plant, both psychoactive and native to South America's Amazon basin. For research on hallucinogens in people, DMT has useful characteristics. Clinically, intravenous DMT is an ultrashort-acting drug. People feel its effects in less than a minute, it peaks within five

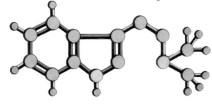

DMT

minutes, and the whole thing is over in less than 30 minutes. In the United States, people who take DMT usually snort it or smoke it with parsley leaves—it doesn't work if you take it orally. You can also inject it (ow).

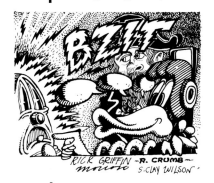

Aside from the ultrashort-acting feature, DMT does all the things you expect from hallucinogens: it changes emotional, perceptual, cognitive, physical and other functions; generates visual and auditory illusions and distortions; causes emotional states to shift and polarize; distorts physical experience; gives novelty and meaning to otherwise mundane thoughts; and can interfere with the ability to interact socially.

DMT: THE EARLY DAYS

In 1956, Stephen Szára was an organic chemist with a medical degree, and chief of the biochemical research at a psychiatric hospital in Budapest. At the

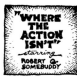

time, Hungary was occupied by Russian Communists. Szára had been interested in psychedelics, especially LSD, since he'd first read about them—mainly in Western books and journals he ordered and read secretly, including *The Doors of Perception,* British author Aldous Huxley's account of his first mescaline trip.

The same year, Szára requested a supply of LSD for research from Sandoz in Basel, Switzerland. Sandoz declined because they didn't want to give the Communists access to LSD, so Szára went back to the lab and synthesized a compound called DMT that he thought might have had LSD-like effects. He followed the leads of researchers who'd isolated the compound in the early 1950s from hallucinogenic snuff powders that South American Indians and Haitians used in religious ceremonies. He tested the DMT on himself and it *was* psychedelic. The effects were like LSD's but lasted 30 to 60 minutes, not nine to 12 hours. Then Szára started his research.

Several months later, the people of Budapest revolted and, for a while, took their streets back from the Communists. Szára remembers the day he decided to leave and find work in the United States: "A colleague... had an uncle who lived near the border and could smuggle us out. He said we could go the day after tomorrow [Nov. 25, 1956]. I went to see my brother and told him I'm going to leave, then did certain things —like making sure that in the hospital I leave

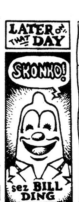
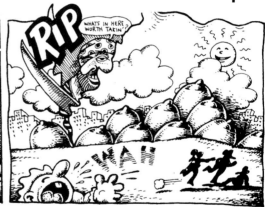

nothing so they cannot trace me. I disposed of certain papers and letters and, at home, anything I thought might be incriminating. We knew leaving was risky but we decided it was worth the risk to have freedom.

"I took with me two little vials of DMT and DET [diethyltryptamine, a psychoactive DMT derivative]. I took my two diplomas, English and German dictionaries, whatever I could wear, an extra shirt, a change of underwear, a heavy overcoat and a couple of sandwiches, all in a briefcase."

They traveled light because they had to walk three miles to cross the border. On the other side, English drivers in Jeeps took them to a safe place in Austria, then to a place where refugees were processed. While Szára was in Vienna, he looked up a researcher he knew was investigating LSD.

"I told him, *If you want to do some work with DMT, I would like to try LSD*. They had an experimental project that involved LSD and they made me a member of the study. I got to try it and they studied me. I didn't like LSD because it lasted too long. I took it about 8 a.m. By about 3 p.m., I was told I can go and I went to the room I was using at the hospital. At 7 p.m. I went to the dining hall where the refugees were having dinner. It was a huge hall with a big white wall on the other side. I looked at the white wall and saw things moving on the wall. I thought, I am not back yet. The walls were breathing."

Before he came to the United States, Szára visited his sister in Berlin, where he was invited to a scientific meeting in Milan and presented a paper on DMT. In Italy Szára ran into a colleague he'd worked with in Budapest who "had brought out [from Budapest] a little brown box I had in the lab. It was full of test tubes [all containing DMT derivatives Szára synthesized but hadn't had time to analyze] and gave it to me in Italy. He was a co-worker so he knew that I would probably like to have it."

In 1957, Szára took a job in the United States with the National Institutes of Health. In 1991, he retired as Biomedical Branch chief of the Preclinical Research Division—part of NIDA— for the Alcohol, Drug Abuse and Mental Health Administration. When I met him in 1987, he still had the brown box full of test tubes, faded labels peeling, half full of 40-year-old, powdery DMT derivatives. "Some of these," he said, poking among the glass tubes, "might be hallucinogenic."

OSCAR JANIGER, LSD & CREATIVITY[82]

LSD was used everywhere in Hollywood and Beverly Hills during the late 1950s, especially on the couches of psychiatrists who treated the stars. Cary Grant took LSD in a session with Dr. Mortimer Hartman, then again with Dr. Oscar Janiger. Therapeutic studies in the 1950s opened new areas of investigation for psychiatrists; one approach was to use LSD to explore creativity. Janiger, the first psychiatrist in the U.S. to clinically investigate DMT, had patients who reported vivid aesthetic perceptions during LSD therapy that they said boosted their appreciation of the arts. One subject compared an acid trip to four years in art school, and urged Janiger to give other artists LSD. This led to a 1955 experiment with Sandoz Pharmaceutical Corp.

▶ THE EXPERIMENT[83]

Janiger started a clinical project to examine LSD's effect on creativity. He asked 100 artists to draw and paint a decorative, colorful Deer Kachina doll before and an hour after taking LSD. An art history professor analyzed the paintings to measure LSD's impact on artistic creativity. During the experiment, typical changes included:

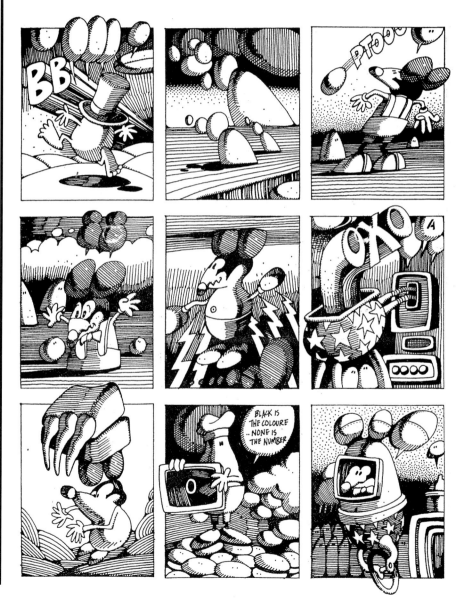

⊚ Relative size expansion: Figures tended to fill all available space and escape its borders.

⊚ Involution: Objects shrunk or filled less space; they got smaller or were imbedded in a matrix.

⊚ Altered figure/ground or a circular viewpoint.

⊚ Altered boundaries: Objects tended to merge with their surroundings; there was less difference between object and subject.

⊚ Movement: Objects or environment continually moved and were more vibrant and emotional.

⊚ More intense color and light.

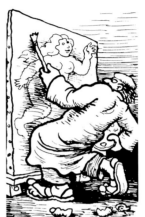

⊚ Oversimplification: Artist eliminated detail and extraneous elements.

⊚ Artist showed objects as symbols or essences.

⊚ Artist showed objects as abstractions.

⊚ Work was fragmented, disorganized, distorted.

LOTS OF ARTISTS THOUGHT their LSD art was aesthetically better than their usual work. The analysis suggested tentatively that the work done on LSD was more interesting on a sensational level, but it wasn't immediately clear the artist produced aesthetically superior work. In most cases, artists kept an imprint of their aesthetic preferences, especially in color and technical facility. Where technical proficiency was lacking before taking LSD, the artist seemed to gain confidence, maybe because of freedom that came from the LSD experience.

"Whether or not the LSD increased creativity is an open question," Janiger's study concluded. "Certainly no systematic research to date has been available to help find an answer. All that can be really be said about the effect of hallucinogens on the creative process is that a strong subjective feeling of creativeness is part of many LSD experiences."[84]

IN THE LATE '50s, Dr. Sidney Cohen, chief of psychosomatic medicine at the Los Angeles Veterans Administration Hospital, surveyed 44 U.S. and Canadian psychiatrists who used LSD therapeutically. They gave him data on 5,000 patients who'd collectively taken more than 25,000 doses of LSD or mescaline. Patient unmanageability was the most common complaint. Of 25,000 cases, there were only eight reports of psychotic reaction that lasted more than 48 hours. LSD therapy didn't kill anyone or turn them into addicts. These and other findings prompted Cohen to report that "with proper precautions, psychedelics are safe when given [under medical supervision] to a selected, healthy group."[85]

THE BEATS

In 1959, beat poet Allen Ginsberg took LSD for the first time at the Mental Research Institute in Palo Alto, California. Like many other beat generation poets and artists, he'd taken peyote several times. The insights of the Beats became poetry and prose. Sometimes they tripped together in small groups and later discussed the best approach to psychedelic sessions. Ginsberg compared their psychedelic expeditions to "being part of a cosmic conspiracy... to resurrect a lost art or a lost knowledge or a lost consciousness."[86]

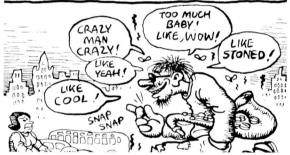

During the grim Cold War, the Beats used hallucinogens to seek visions, abandon an unbearable world and tap their own mind power. Drugs fueled their rebellion against conformity. They sneered at the seekers after success, cleanliness and THINGS. The Beats took on what the masses rejected: jazz, marijuana, Buddhist meditation, their faster-than-a-speeding-bullet lifestyle

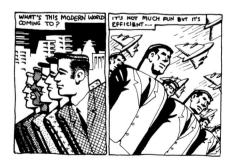

and a hunger for sensation. The Beats defied the robotic '50s by going antisocial; urging the next generation on to psychological freedom from convention and the inevitable experiments with drugs: "The Beats saw psychedelics as truth drugs that enhanced creative independence. They were open about their drug use, and beat literature flow[ed] from intoxicated states."[87]

As cultural expatriates and inveterate wave-riders, the Beats paddled out on psychedelic long-boards to wait for The Big One. Far behind them, because of them, one massive oceanic plate slid slowly under another. The motion set off a seismic spectrum of long-period swells, ending in a massive tidal wave—a tsunami. As the 1950s slid 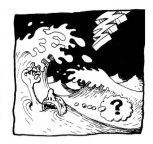 slowly under the 1960s, hallucinogens created a swell of nonconformity that

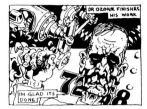 grew into a mass rebellion and moved like a wall toward the next decade.[88]

Down the coast, beach-dwellers shaded their eyes and squinted at the rising sea. But, as seismologists like to say, by the time you can see a tsunami coming, it's too late.

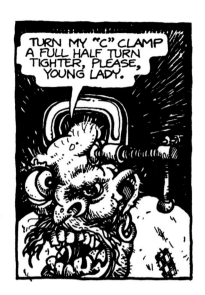

Chapter 5

THE 1960s: LSD — OUT OF KILTER WITH THE BASIC ASSUMPTIONS OF WESTERN MEDICINE

"A great deal of intelligence can be invested in ignorance when the need for illusion is deep."—Saul Bellow [89]

REGULATION, RESTRICTION & A LITTLE RESEARCH

In 1960, Dr. Sidney Cohen of UCLA and the Veteran's Hospital in Los Angeles published findings on adverse reactions to LSD based on a survey of 5,000 people and 25,000 acid trips. Of 1,000 ingestions, he counted 1.8 psychotic episodes, 1.2 attempted suicides and 0.4 completed suicides. Cohen concluded that LSD was "an astonishingly safe drug," and this led to a boom in LSD psychotherapy over the next two years. In 1961, the late great Daniel X. Freedman, Yale University psychiatry professor and hallucinogen researcher, was first to examine LSD's effects on serotonin metabolism. But it was 1961 and, as a field, the neurosciences were still pretty primeval, technologically speaking.

Researchers knew there was serotonin in the brain but they didn't know where. They knew it was part of the brain's electrochemical communication network of nerve cells (neurons). And they could measure serotonin levels in the whole brain or brain regions, but no one knew what it did there. What Freedman found in 1961 was that after exposure to LSD, brain serotonin levels rose.

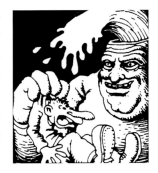

HIGHLIGHTS: LSD & MENTAL HEALTH

Meanwhile, back in the real world, U.S. psychiatrists were starting to understand that LSD might do something for alcoholics and other 'mental' patients who got no help from conventional psychotherapy.

 SPRING GROVE[90]

In 1963, researchers started working with patients hospitalized at Spring Grove State Hospital in Baltimore. As part of its research program, Spring Grove conducted a series of well-designed studies using LSD therapy to treat chronic alcoholics, severe neurotics and terminal cancer patients. The National Institute of Mental Health (NIMH) funded the project with more than $4 million. Psychiatrists Walter Pahnke and later Stanislav Grof headed the research team.

An 18-month follow-up investigation of active and placebo groups showed no difference between them. Drinking behavior data confirmed this.

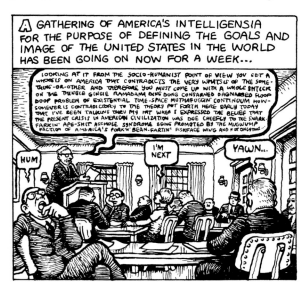

After four weeks of preparatory psychotherapy, even people who took the active placebo showed improved drinking behavior. That meant the effect of high-dose LSD related to the immediate success of 51 percent of patients, but not to the follow-up period. LSD helped, at least in the short term.

▸ "AN ALIBI FOR KICKS..."

In 1966, hearings convened hastily in Washington to deal with what people increasingly saw as the growing LSD problem. At a hearing of the Senate subcommittee on juvenile delinquency, Chairman Senator Thomas Dodd dismissed "consciousness expansion as an alibi for kicks" and proposed strict new laws aimed at the "pseudo-intellectuals" who advocated drug use. Scientists, health officials and law enforcement experts said people who independently used LSD for nonmedical purposes became psychotic, violent and likely to use more dangerous drugs.[91]

In May 1966, Senator Robert Kennedy opened hearings before the Senate subcommittee on executive reorganization. The committee wanted to examine the government's ability to deal with LSD research and regulation, and the federal response to LSD-related problems.

The hearing featured an all-star line-up of premier LSD researchers, including Sidney Cohen, M.D., chief of psychosomatic medicine for the Los Angeles VA Hospital; Daniel X. Freedman, M.D., a Yale University psychiatry professor and researcher; Timothy Leary, Ph.D.,* then-president of the Castalia Foundation for Psychedelic Research (represented by Larry Bogart of New York's Conservation Center); and Stanley Yolles, M.D., from the National Institute of Mental Health (NIMH). Also attending were FDA Commissioner James Goddard, M.D., and General Counsel William Goodrich; Richard Blum, Ph.D., consultant to the President's Commission on Law Enforcement and Administration of

---

*1920-1996. God rest his Day Glo® soul. Visit Timothy Leary's home page on the Internet @ http://www.leary.com.

1962: THE GOOD FRIDAY EXPERIMENT

On Good Friday in 1962, psychiatrist Walter Pahnke did an experiment to determine whether psilocybin could help people have something like mystical religious experiences. Maybe it helped that before entering medical school he'd earned a doctor of divinity degree. The experiment involved 20 theology students who said they'd had mystical religious experiences. They all took a drug Pahnke said was psilocybin. But 10 got psilocybin and 10 got nicotinic acid, a B vitamin that makes the skin feel warm and tingly—also a minor side effect of psilocybin. Three of 10 students who took psilocybin had profound mystical experiences. None of the 10 on nicotinic acid had them.

—from *Drugs and the Brain* by Solomon Snyder, M.D., p.183–184

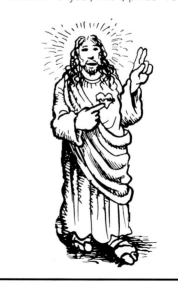

Justice; and Philip Lee, M.D., assistant secretary for Health and Scientific Affairs at the Department of Health, Education & Welfare (now the Department of Health and Human Services or DHHS).

"Experiments indicate LSD may be useful in treating alcoholics," Kennedy told the subcommittee. "It has been helpful...as an adjunct to psychotherapy for mentally ill people. If we in the federal government allow legitimate uses to be interfered with, the loss to the nation of potential aid for the handicapped would be serious. If LSD has slipped away from us, other new discoveries might be misused and social dangers created because we pay too little attention to the interlocking design for our programs."

Goddard of the FDA, which in 1966 had jurisdiction over LSD, described LSD's public abuse and resulting psychiatric problems, criminal investigations, and illegal production and distribution. The FDA put LSD at the top of

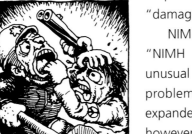

its priority list of drug-abuse targets because it "damages the mind power of young Americans."

NIMH's Yolles called for more LSD research. "NIMH clearly recognizes that LSD presents... unusual research opportunities and an abuse problem. Both areas require continued and expanded research effort," he said. "The drug, however, is important for [understanding] brain function and behavior, and as a potentially powerful therapeutic tool and, as such, supplies should be available to responsible investigators."

Like Goddard and other witnesses, Yolles proposed that the feds distribute public information emphasizing the potential dangers of hallucinogens, amphetamines and barbiturates. Health and Scientific Affairs' Lee testified that LSD was dangerous, but that LSD research by competent investigators should continue.

In written testimony, Leary proposed forming a national commission of psychiatrists, social scientists and religious leaders, and representatives from the arts, the drug industry, law enforcement and government regulatory agencies to develop a broad LSD research and abuse control program. He said the commission could develop a licensing procedure so responsible, healthy adults could use LSD for self-understanding, and that LSD should be administered only in psychedelic training centers where experienced guides could screen, prepare, and guide the applicants.

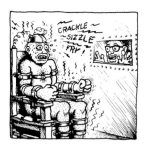

Stan Yolles said taking LSD without medical supervision was risky, but making possession a crime would encourage its use and drive it underground. Instead he called for a program of education and prevention.

Senator Jacob Javits said an education program would be more effective combined with prohibitions on possession. Yolles disagreed. "We are dealing with a different class of compound [than heroin or narcotics]," he told Javits. "A few exposures to narcotics and continued use of them leads to physical addiction. [LSD] is a different story. One or two doses may be all the student ever uses. If we make this a crime, we may find we are filling up our jails with a bunch of college students."

AFTER THE INITIAL RUSH of success with hallucinogens in psychotherapeutic and scientific research, LSD in the early '60s was practically on its way to the drug store. Then something went horribly wrong. In 1967 there was a little progress in research and lots of progress in regulation. Daniel Freedman found that exposure to LSD caused levels of a major serotonin metabolite, 5-hydroxyindoleacetic acid (5-HIAA), to drop. That's more than anyone knew before, but it still didn't explain serotonin's role or its relationship to LSD. Then researcher Albert Cohen and colleagues Marinello and Bach published an article in *Science*, the

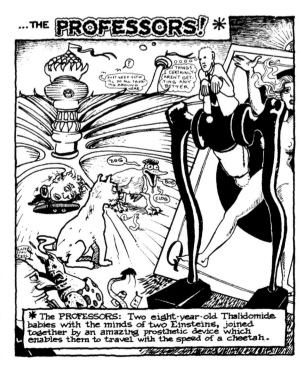

* The PROFESSORS: Two eight-year-old Thalidomide babies with the minds of two Einsteins, joined together by an amazing prosthetic device which enables them to travel with the speed of a cheetah.

NEWSPAPER HEADLINES, 1966-69[*]

Students Use Labs for Making LSD New York, April 1966

Plunge Kills Coed; LSD Is Suspected Berkeley, February 1967

Doctor Lists Gains With LSD Therapy Baltimore, March 1967

Banana Smokers Say It's Like Pot Washington, D.C., March 1967

Hippies Find Ways to Avoid Working San Francisco, April 1967

Japanese Hippies Take Over a Park in Tokyo Tokyo, April 1967

25 Arrested in Raid At 'Psychedelic' House Washington, D.C., May 1967

LSD-Leukemia Link Suspected Oregon, May 1967

6 Seized; LSD Ring Believed Uncovered San Diego, July 1967

LSD... STP... What's Next for Hippies? Los Angeles, July 1967

FDA Identifies STP, Warns of Danger in Use Washington, D.C., July 1967

Chromosome Break Seen in LSD Users' Children Oregon, September 1967

Military Is Studying the Use of Marijuana by GIs in Vietnam
Saigon, September 1967

Today's Runaways Head for Hippie Habitats Hollywood, September 1967

Summer's End: A Bad Trip San Francisco, September 1967

Cool Salesmen Create a Vast Dope Market San Francisco, October 1967

NY Jury Acquits LSD 'Tripper' in Murder of Kin October 1967

3-Month-Old Hippie Clinic in San Francisco Closes
San Francisco, October 1967

House Unit Backs a Bill to Penalize Possession of LSD
Washington, D.C., November 1967

LSD Held No Help to Alcoholics Canada, November 1967

Army Makes 'Pot' For Use in Warfare
Buffalo, New York, February 1969

City Test of Cheap Drug Set for Heroin Addicts Washington, D.C., February 1969

Nixon Orders War on Drug Peddling Washington, D.C., February 1969

Heroin Invades the White Middle Class Reston, Virginia, February 1969

Few Students are Really Acidheads Connecticut, March 1969

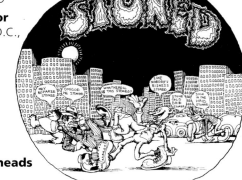

[*]From a collection of original newspaper articles compiled by Dr. Stephen Szára, Biomedical Branch chief (ret.), Preclinical Research Division at the former Alcohol, Drug Abuse and Mental Health Administration, part of NIDA in Bethesda, Maryland. Used with permission.

journal of the American Association for the Advancement of Science, claiming that LSD caused chromosome damage in human leukocyte cells.

Around the same time, the *Saturday Evening Post* used an LSD caption under a photo of deformed babies born to mothers who had taken a chemically flawed morning-sickness drug called Thalidomide.[92] It didn't take the print and broadcast media long to spew the gruesome misinformation into every American living room. And before other researchers could say, *Let's check out this data,* people around the country who knew nothing else thought they knew that LSD damaged genetic material and produced deformed babies, among other things, none of which, as it turns out, was true.

THE MARYLAND PSYCHIATRIC RESEARCH CENTER[93]

In 1968, research at the Maryland Psychiatric Research Center (MPRC) picked up where Spring Grove left off and continued until 1976, when the Maryland state government made a political decision to end psychedelic research. But from 1968 to 1976, researchers at MPRC investigated the usefulness of psychedelic psychotherapy with alcoholics, neurotics, drug addicts and terminally ill patients. NIMH funded the double-blind, controlled studies of alcoholics and neurotics. In 1971, Albert Kurland, M.D., and colleagues published results of their psychedelic studies on 175 chronic alcoholics. Treatment included one high-dose LSD session. To prepare for the 8- to 10-hour

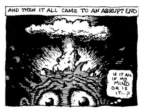
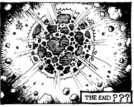

LSD session, patients spent four intense weeks in psychotherapy. During the LSD session, therapists helped patients have transcendental experiences. Statistics showed that 70 percent of patients had peak experiences. The double-blind study used 150 mcg of LSD as an active placebo for controls, and 300-500 mcg for treatment.

SCIENCE & PSYCHEDELICS

STEPHAN SZÁRA

In 1968, Stephen Szára, M.D., D.Sc., was chief of the Psycho-pharmacology Section in the NIMH Clinical Psychopharmacology lab at St. Elizabeth's Hospital in Washington, D.C. He'd studied psychedelics for decades and in 1956 had discovered hallucinogenic activity in a series of tryptamine derivatives,

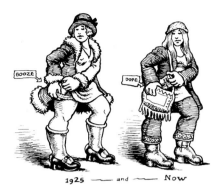

BOOZE DOPE

1925 ———— and ———— Now

including DMT. Later he supervised and participated in more than 100 administrations of the drugs to research volunteers.

In January that year, Szára's director asked him to visit San Francisco, Los Angeles and New York to study the hippie movement and the role of hallucinogens in psychedelic cults. He was supposed to talk to doctors, psychologists and sociologists, and record personal impressions as he visited the psychedelic shops, coffee houses, paraphernalia shops, psychedelic theaters and meditation rooms of Haight Street in San Francisco, Telegraph Avenue in Berkeley, Sunset Strip in Hollywood, N. Fairfax Avenue in Los Angeles, St. Mark's Place in New York's East Village, MacDougal Street in the West Village, and M Street and Dupont Circle in Washington, D.C. He was also asked to verify media stories on hippies and drug use; formulate scientific hypotheses on the biochemical, psychological or social mechanisms involved; and suggest research approaches for related public health problems.

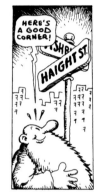

HERE'S A GOOD CORNER!

HAIGHT ST.

Szára originally intended to contact psychiatrist friends and interview their drug-using patients. Then he realized that drugs were an important but small part of the hippie culture—the picture he'd get this way would be like learning about the car's role in America by going to hospitals and interviewing accident victims. It would ignore positive aspects of the culture that might be important. Because he only had four days in each city, he decided to meet a few psychiatrists, psychologists and sociologists, and see as much of the psychedelic culture as possible. He also kept an eye on hippies in his own area, Washington, D.C., during the summer of 1967. His report included personal observations and experiences, interviews and samples of each city's underground press offerings.

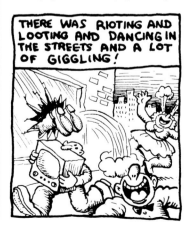

THERE WAS RIOTING AND LOOTING AND DANCING IN THE STREETS AND A LOT OF GIGGLING!

He defined hippies as "people who have subjective feelings of being aware of reality and all that is taking place about them in nature, life and society; and who seek a better world where an ethic of indi-

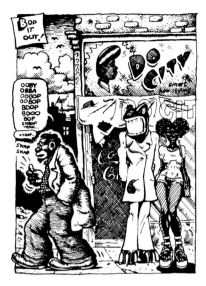

vidual freedom, love and personal honesty prevails."* This definition didn't include pseudohippies—hangers-on who secretly got money from home but lived in hip communities, grew long hair, wore psychedelic clothes and identified with the action but had no serious commitment to the hippie ethic and its social consequences.

Szára believed drugs like LSD, marijuana and DMT were critical to producing the subjective feelings of awareness that changed people's value systems and prompted them to join the hippie movement and seek a better world. Magazines and newspapers stressed the hippies' almost exclusive white, middle-class origin, but Szára found hippies in integrated communities that reflected a local area's ethnic population. He also found that drug use among hippies was the biggest public concern and caused most legal, medical, psychological and social problems, and confirmed media reports of widespread illegal drug use by hippies in every city he visited.

LSD was a major drug on the hippie scene. All black-market LSD was produced illegally (Sandoz LSD was no longer available) and he found a big variation in the quality of [street] acid. 'Owsley's acid' was considered the best quality, but after police raids it tended to get replaced by poorer-quality LSD, often mixed with methedrine (speed). Conservative estimates of the Haight acid market were 200,000 doses a month at $2 and $2.50 each.

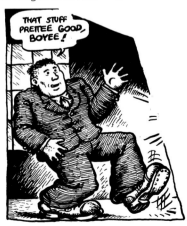

DMT had a minor role in the hippie movement. It was available but more expensive than LSD. Users smoked it as dried, DMT-soaked parsley leaves. It was called the "businessman's lunchtime psychedelic" because the intense high lasted less than an hour. When Szára visited southern California, it seemed significant to

*From Stephen Szára, M.D., D.Sc., "A Scientist Looks at the Hippies," an unpublished report to his supervisor in the Psychopharmacology Section, National Institute on Mental Health, Clinical Psychopharmacology lab, St. Elizabeth's Hospital, after visiting Haight-Ashbury and other hippie neighborhoods around the country (Washington, D.C., 1968). Used with permission.

him that the grocery store in Topanga Canyon, a small rural community near Los Angeles, was doing a brisk business in dried parsley leaves.

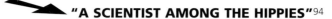

"A SCIENTIST AMONG THE HIPPIES"[94]

From Szára's report: Sunday night, Avalon Ballroom, San Francisco, 1968

"The ballroom is dimly lit and has projection screens on three walls around the room," Szára wrote in a 1968 report that wouldn't be published until 1997 (right here in *Trips*). "A dozen slide projectors project abstract color patterns, faces or pictures of statues or paintings, usually of a religious character. Superimposed on the changing patterns are dancing patterns from six overhead liquid-projectors.

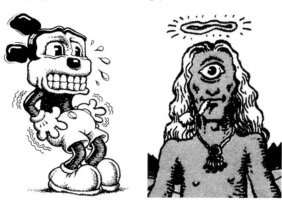
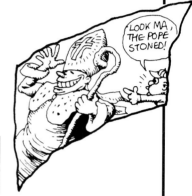

"These project images from large watchglasses filled with an oil-water mixture, dyed with color, and moved by hand or by another watchglass on the liquid's surface. This creates amoeba-like images that move to the music. In some corners of the screens are looped projections of short sequences from old movies, Mickey Mouse cartoons, or real or animated sexually suggestive scenes. Another visual stimulus is a flickering strobe light, under which the dancing people seem mechanized, their movements jerky as in old-time movies.

"Music called acid rock is played continuously by two or three orchestras alternating with each other. It is called acid rock because many song lyrics allude to LSD and pot, and because it employs a monotonous, harshly amplified drone-like sound that can act as a psychedelic stimulus. In the midst of a routine rock-and-roll number, for instance, the players may focus on a particular pattern that they repeat again and again, louder and louder until the limit of the human eardrum is reached, then suddenly stops.

"Only part of the audience actually dances on the floors. A large portion of youngsters (mostly teenaged girls) lie in front of the screens and orchestra, practically 'stoned' under the barrage of visual and auditory bombardments. I saw similar

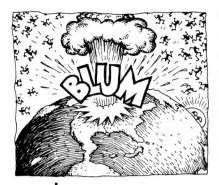

arrangements and happenings at Magic Mushrooms and Genesis IX in Los Angeles, at the Electric Circus in New York, and at the Ambassador Theater in Washington, D.C. I describe these experiences in detail because acid rock music seems an essential part of the hippie scene and is likely to be the main carrier of the psychedelic message into the future, even if the hippie subculture as we know it today passes.

"The audiences at these shows are not typical hippies (they could not afford the whopping $3.50 to $4.50 admission fee), but college and high school kids can afford it. This is significant because they, with their higher educational development, might be more successful in formulating a convincing social philosophy and integrating the psychedelic experience with ongoing life.

"One result of drugs like LSD is that a tremendous array of possibilities present themselves that first overwhelm the subject, then give a powerful subjective feeling of freedom in terms of available choices. Since the tradition of culture has suppressed most of these possibilities, it is understandable that an impatience with traditional ways and values arises and a revolutionary, rebellious attitude emerges. A long way lies ahead in creating and disseminating information through research and education before intelligent decisions can be assured at the individual level. In the meantime, widespread illegal and mostly uncontrolled use of psychedelic drugs create some nonmedical problems. A subtle rearrangement of these young people's subjective value system might remain and play a part in future decisions that affect the individuals and society. The drug movement's impact can best be seen within the changing value system, and it is very hard to predict the effect it may have on the final outcome of the hippie movement and on the future of established society."

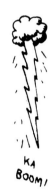

IN 1968, LESS THAN two years after the Senate LSD hearings, Public Law 639 amended the Federal Food, Drug and Cosmetic Act to increase the penalties for unlawful acts involving LSD. In 1970, the Comprehensive Drug Abuse Prevention and Control Act combined PL 639, the Harrison Narcotics Act of 1914, the Marijuana Tax Act of 1937 and every other drug law passed since the turn of the century into one massive drug law, called the Controlled Substances Act.[94]

In a way, the feds themselves instigated the chemical chaos of the '60s and turned the paranoid drug legislation into the most restrictive, least obeyed series of laws since 55 mph speed limits on the interstates. Back then, if regular citizens even glanced at a picture of the guys who isolated the active principles in marijuana or LSD, they went straight to jail for as long as anyone could hold them. The only people exempt from the law in this area were those who spent the '50s and half the '60s, that we know about, professionally abusing drugs, drug laws and the constitutional rights of fellow citizens. Because, "as it turns out, nearly every drug that hit the black market during the 1960s—marijuana, cocaine, heroin, PCP, amyl nitrate, mushrooms, DMT, barbiturates, laughing gas, speed—had...been scrutinized," tested on whoever was handy, and, "in some cases, refined by CIA and Army scientists."[96]

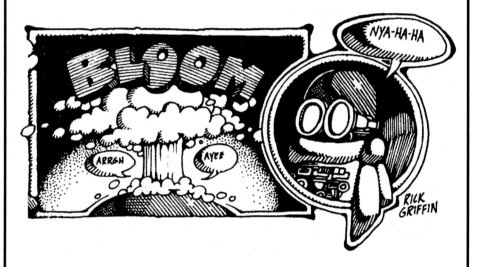

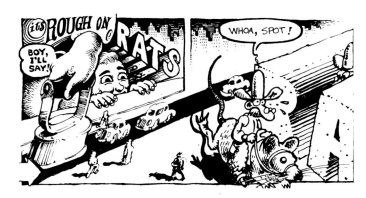

Chapter 6

1970–1990: ANIMAL PHARM—ROUGH ON RATS

THERE WAS ONLY ONE THING WRONG with human hallucinogen research from about 1970 to 1991—it wasn't happening, especially in
the United States. So hallucinogen researchers studied the drugs in the next
best thing—animals. Over the years, mice, rats, monkeys, cats, dogs, rabbits,
bees and spiders took more drugs than Keith *Richards*[97] so scientists could
figure out how neurotransmitters, receptors and
hallucinogens actually worked in brain systems.
When the drug epidemic finally hits the animal and
insect kingdoms, researchers will be *ready.*

DRUG DISCRIMINATION, ANIMALS & HALLUCINOGENS

But really. What can they learn from rats? One way
researchers use animals to study the subjective and
behavioral effects of drugs is drug discrimination. In this model, a scientist
trains a rat or whatever to press different levers in a test chamber when it:

1. feels the effects of a specific dose of a training drug like LSD,
2. recognizes a different dose of the same training drug,
3. feels the effects of a different drug, or
4. gets a saline solution that has no effects.

THAT'S DRUG DISCRIMINATION—when an animal recognizes or discriminates among the effects of the training drug and the other drugs and saline solution. That's how researchers test a new drug—by giving it to a rat that's trained

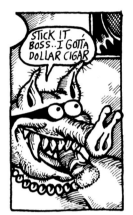

to recognize one drug, and seeing which lever the rat presses. If the rat presses the training-drug lever, the new drug probably feels like the training drug. If the rat presses the saline-solution lever, the new drug probably feels different from the training drug.

Drug discrimination helps scientists classify new drugs and answer questions like how long it takes the drug to start working, how long it lasts, how it works, whether it's like other drugs, how it breaks down in the body, the relationship between the drug's chemical structure and the behavior it causes, and what other drugs (antagonists) might reverse its effects—without actually taking the drugs themselves.[98] Most researchers use test chambers with two levers, but some tests use three-lever chambers.

Researchers like to use rats, pigeons and monkeys in drug discrimination, but they're starting to use other animals and people, even though people aren't as good at it as animals.[99] So animals are useful in the lab—to a point. The problem with psychedelics and animal research, says Dr. Geraline Lin, program officer in the Basic Research Division at NIDA, "is that with psychedelics you're talking about mental activity. With pain, for instance, you can have an animal model that's not 100 percent but it's quite reasonable and can be translated to the human [nervous system].

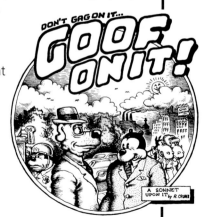

"When you talk about mental activity... [animal] reactions are supposed to reflect human reactions, but who knows? An animal gives indirect information. Only human beings can tell you how they feel. Until you get data from humans, you always have a gap. In a lot of studies that's true, but especially for mental activity. In drug discrimination," she adds, "some cue in the animal prompts it to make a certain response, but we still don't know what that means.

"It's very important that preclinical [in the lab] and clinical [with people] studies complement each other. You need to see if what you find in animals is actually what happens in humans. You have to apply what 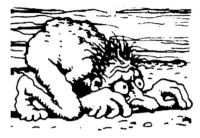 you learn from animals to the human study design, then check these results back against the animal data, then back and forth, back and forth. The purpose of all animal studies, all the research, is to apply the knowledge to humans. If you can never apply it to humans, you don't need animal studies. That's the basic principle in all areas of research and it should apply in [the hallucinogen] area, too... The final answer—actually for all research but acutely in this area—the bottom line is the human being."

 RICHARD GLENNON SEZ

From a February 1996 interview with Richard A. Glennon, Ph.D., professor of medicinal chemistry, Department of Medicinal Chemistry, Medical College of Virginia School of Pharmacy, Virginia Commonwealth University, Richmond.

"I think drug discrimination has been a boon to CNS [central nervous system] medicinal chemistry. Certainly the area of research on hallucinogenic agents wouldn't be able to survive without it. When we published back in the early 1980s a correlation between drug discrimination and hallucinogenic potency, that clinched it—that we were looking at something that could be very useful. It was tough, 10 or 15 years ago, trying to get this stuff published. You had to argue with the reviewers. Now it's an accepted technique. It may not be a model of hallucinogenic activity, we've never said it is, but it's giving us the kind of information we want, qualitatively and quantitatively, about compounds known to be hallucinogenic in humans. If you listen carefully, you'll realize we've never once said the animals are hallucinating. Never ever. We have no idea what's going on in their heads. There are a lot of animal models for hallucinogenic activity, but none are foolproof. Drug discrimination is probably the closest we'll come to identifying what's going on.

"If you have animals trained to recognize a specific hallucinogen, drug discrimination can be used to ask questions of the animals who are given a new drug—

maybe something you've found out on the street, something the DEA sent you, or compounds we synthesize to find out what parts of the molecule are important for [drug] activity. We administer these to the animal and they'll either recognize it or not. The questions we can ask are, Does it produce the same effect as the drug the animal is trained to recognize? If so, how potent is it? If they recognize it, they'll tell us how potent it is compared to what they were trained to recognize. They tell us behaviorally, by the responses they make [during the drug tests]."

IN THE EARLY 1980s, Glennon's lab started work on MDA, a mild hallucinogen that passed through the CIA's clandestine street-drug distribution program and got popular in the late '60s as the 'hug drug' because of its mellow effects. But in Richard Glennon's lab, MDA was sort of a trick compound for the drug discrimination rats because it's an isomer. Isomers are chemically identical compounds that are oriented differently in space. Like on *Star Trek: The Next Generation,* when some space anomaly gives Data an evil twin. Data's evil twin holds the Enterprise hostage; MDA's *R(-)* and *S(+)* isomers rotate polarized light in opposite directions and give the compounds different chemical properties.

"The drug discrimination studies showed that the hallucinogenic activity of MDA was likely associated with its R(-)isomer; this confirmed what had been previously shown to be the case in humans. Drug discrimination also showed that the S(+)isomer of MDA was an amphetamine-like stimulant. It was proposed that the dual hallucinogenic/stimulant actions of racemic MDA, then, represented the combined effect of the hallucinogenic R(-)isomer and the stimulant S(+)isomer." Glennon's drug discrimination tests confirmed that.

"We had looked at many different hallucinogens as possible training drugs (e.g. 5-methoxy-N,N-dimethyltryptamine, LSD) but ultimately found that the phenylisopropylamine hallucinogen DOM* was best for the kinds of things we wanted to do." We didn't know why at the time, now we do—it's quite selective [has a narrow range of effects]. LSD was [pharmacologically] dirty, meaning it had lots of different effects that were too hard to follow. We might be looking at a side effect and not know it. Our LSD-trained animals recognized hallucinogens but they recognized a lot of other stuff too.

"To the untrained eye, these structures have more similarities than differences. DOM is what's called a phenylisopropylamine. Amphetamine is also a phenylisopropy-

---

*Chemist Alexander Shulgin developed DOM in the 1960s when he worked as a researcher for Dow Chemical Co. Chemically it's 2,5-dimethoxy-4-methylamphetamine, called STP in the '60s (which either stood for serenity, tranquility and peace, or for the gas additive STP). Shulgin juggled the methoxy groups and added a methyl group to make it 50 to 100 times more potent than mescaline, which is pretty weak. Who says chemistry isn't fun?

lamine, but amphetamine is a stimulant and DOM is a hallucinogen... We wanted to classify all these phenylisopropylamines as hallucinogen-like or amphetamine-like. We had DOM-trained animals and amphetamine-trained animals, and we looked at 200 or 300 different compounds in all of them. It took us 10 or 12 years. "In this manner, we have been able to classify phenylisopropylamines (and other agents) as being either DOM-like, amphetamine-like, or like neither. We found the same thing with

DOM

alpha-ethyltryptamine or, as it is known on the street, "ET." One isomer is DOM-like, one is amphetamine-like, and the racemate is recognized by MDMA-trained animals. But the one drug both groups of animals recognized was MDA. So we trained another group of animals to recognize MDA, the idea being that animals trained to recognize racemic MDA [equal parts R(-) and S(+) isomers] should have both effects.

"We expected MDA animals to recognize hallucinogens like DOM and LSD, but they should also recognize stimulants like amphetamine and cocaine. And they did. MDA-trained animals recognized both classes of drugs. What's being used on the street is a racemic mixture [of MDA]. You'd expect that to have hallucinogen-like effects and speed-like effects, but milder forms of both. So it's not very potent in either category but it is active. This supports exactly our animal studies from the 1980s.

"In the mid 1980s we proposed that classical hallucinogens produce their effects by activating a population of neurotransmitter receptors in the brain. More

AMPHETAMINE

specifically, we proposed that these were a type of serotonin receptor called (at that time) the 5-HT$_2$ receptors; today, these receptors are referred to as 5-HT$_{2A}$ receptors. Thus, if hallucinogens work by activating these receptors, administration of 5-HT$_2$ antagonists (agents capable of blocking the receptor and preventing the drug from interacting with it to result in a productive interaction) in combination with a hallucinogen should antagonize or block the effects of the hallucinogen. We demonstrated this in a number of experiments. Extending this to MDA, then, co-administration of 5-HT$_2$ antagonists should block the effect of the hallucinogenic R(-)MDA isomer, but should have no effect on the stimulant S(+)isomer. And that is exactly what happened." Really neat. That took us into MDMA [ecstasy], which is nothing more than the N-methyl analog of MDA.

CLASSICAL AND OTHER HALLUCINOGENS[100]

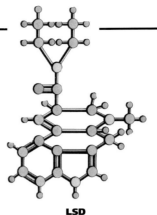

LSD

CLASSICAL HALLUCINOGENS

Indolealkylamine hallucinogens

**Simple tryptamines
(DMT, 5-methoxy-DMT, psilocin)**

Alpha-methyltryptamines

Beta-carbolines (harmine, harmaline)

**Ergolines
(LSD, other lysergic acid analogs)**

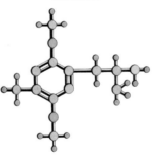

DMT

PHENYLALKYLAMINES

Phenethylamines (mescaline)

Phenylisopropylamines (DOM, DOB)

PSILOCIN

OTHER HALLUCINOGENS

Cannabinoids

Phencyclidine (PCP)-related agents

Certain cholinergic agents

Miscellaneous

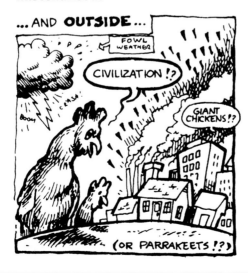

DOM

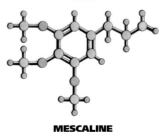

MESCALINE

"If you add an N-methyl group [written CH₃] to a phenylisopropylamine hallucinogen, it dramatically decreases activity. If you take an amphetamine-like stimulant and add a methyl group, that's like going from amphetamine to methamphetamine—increased activity. So if you add an N-methyl group to MDA, which has hallucinogen and amphetamine components, the hallucinogen component should go down, the amphetamine component should go up.

"We expected MDMA to be more of a stimulant than anything else, and there's no question it's a stimulant. But David Nichols [a medicinal chemist and psychopharmacologist at Purdue University] found that MDMA had some other effect as well. Nobody knew what it was, but now it seems to be more of an empathogenic [from the word empathy—understanding someone else's situation or feelings] effect. David Nichols coined the term entactogen (a touching within) because there was a need for a term to separate [MDMA] from the other classes of drugs. David was first to suggest MDMA had a different effect and we had trouble agreeing with that for a long time. But we were first to train animals to MDMA [and they only partially] recognized amphetamine. Something else was going on... So over the last five or seven years, we've come to agree with David that there's something else going on that's unique to this compound... We refer to it as the *other* activity, because we don't know what it is."

Several research groups that have studied the issue cite evidence that the 'other activity' is serotonin release. There's no real consensus yet, but the investigators believe serotonin release is a major component of the action of MDMA.

"Another thing we're looking at now," Glennon says, "are the beta-carbolines like harmaline, found in South America. We were first to train animals to discriminate a beta-carboline hallucinogen [in 1994 but haven't published the results] and now have classified hallucinogens into various categories and trained animals up to an example of each classical hallucinogen.

"In the ergoline family we have LSD-trained animals, in the simple tryptamine family we have 5-methoxy-DMT animals, in the phenylethylamine family we have mescaline-trained animals, in the phenylisopropylamine family we have DOM-trained animals, and in the beta-carboline family we have harmaline.

"The beauty of the classification system is that animals trained to a specific member of one family of classical hallucinogens recognize members from other families of classical hallucinogens. For example, DOM-trained animals recognize LSD, mescaline, and 5-methoxy-N,N-dimethyltryptamine, whereas animals trained to discriminate 5-methoxy-N,N-dimethyltryptamine recognize DOM, LSD, and mescaline, and so on. In essence, this is a fail-safe system because recognition is multidirectional."

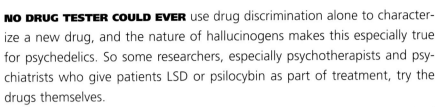

NO DRUG TESTER COULD EVER use drug discrimination alone to characterize a new drug, and the nature of hallucinogens makes this especially true for psychedelics. So some researchers, especially psychotherapists and psychiatrists who give patients LSD or psilocybin as part of treatment, try the drugs themselves.

Stephen Szára—physician, research scientist and retired Biomedical Branch chief of NIDA's Preclinical Research Division—was one of them. As mentioned in Chapter 4, in 1956 at the University of Budapest he isolated dimethyltryptamine (DMT) and tested the drug on lab animals. But this told him nothing about whether the drug was psychoactive. He made himself the first volunteer.[101]

"I took it by mouth...a quarter of a milligram of the substance. I remember, having read [Albert] Hofmann's story, that he took what he thought was a small dose—like .25 mg of LSD—and he really was bombed out. So I decided to start at a very small level. I took .25 mg and nothing happened. Two days later I took a higher dose, and so on. I went up to about 10 mg/kg dose and still nothing happened. For a moment I got discouraged, then somebody suggested that... maybe you have to take it... intramuscularly or intravenously or subcutaneously.

"I... asked my friend at the [hospital] pharmacy department... to prepare a sterile injectable solution of dimethyltryptamine for me. The first small dose, which I injected intramuscularly, was .5 mg/kilo.

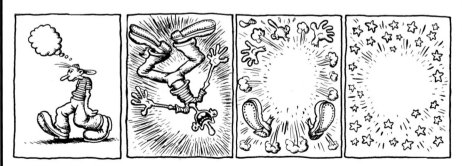

"In 3 or 4 minutes I started to experience visual sensations that were very similar to what I had read in the descriptions by Hofmann [LSD] and [Aldous] Huxley [mescaline].

"I got very, very excited. It was obvious this was the secret... that you would have to give it parenterally, intramuscularly. As I remember it now... I repeated it once again on myself at a slightly higher dose before two of my friends and colleagues volunteered. We were trying to find out whether these effects were... reproducible and [to identify] the parameters involved. Based upon these experiments on ourselves, we developed an evaluation protocol and... decided to test the drug on a number of other subjects."

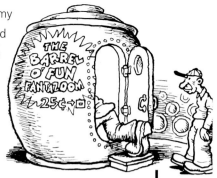

AFTERWARD, SZÁRA STUDIED and worked with DMT and other hallucinogens for nearly 40 years. During a 1987 interview at his NIDA office in Bethesda, Maryland, he tried to explain why self-testing often seems to be part of hallucinogen research.

"Do all drug researchers try the drugs they develop," I asked, "like for hives or heart disease or swollen glands?"

"No," he said. "This drug interferes with the most precious human ability—awareness. It interfered with consciousness and the effect was very strange. No [researchers] were willing to give someone else something they didn't know for themselves was safe. That was the main reason."

Then there was scientific curiosity.

"Everyone was aware that LSD and mescaline would change perception, feeling states and a number of other psychological parameters," he added, "so we anticipated that effect. But the curiosity was primarily scientific."

I said, "You didn't do it for fun, then, like people do now?"

"No," he shook his head. Smiled suddenly. "But we had fun."

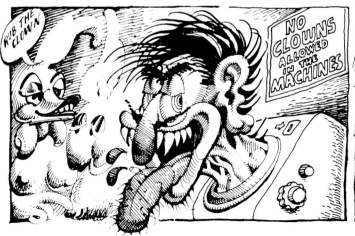

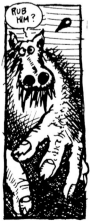

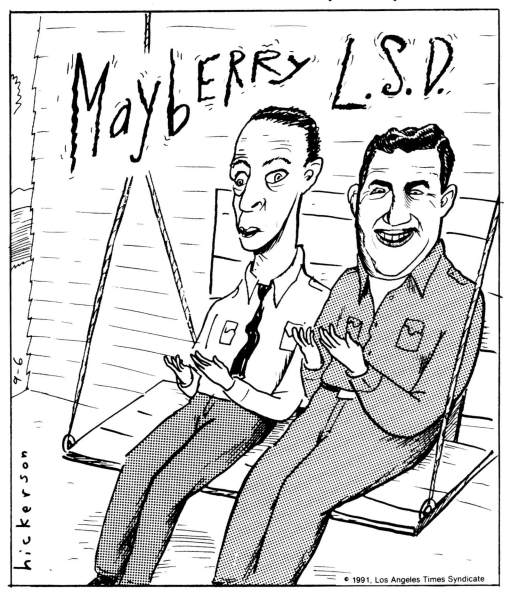

"Hey, Barn... Have you ever REALLY looked at your hands?"

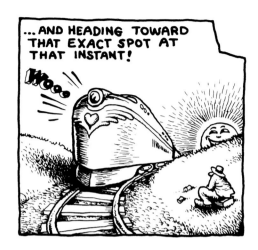

"...AND HEADING TOWARD THAT EXACT SPOT AT THAT INSTANT!"

Woo

Chapter 7

1991-1993: CIVILIZATION HO! [102]

BETWEEN 1991 AND 1993 the field wasn't exactly a blur, but it was moving again, for a couple of reasons. FDA announced in 1992 that it would (stop `beating its wife') treat hallucinogens like any other drug—even though it was never an official policy to do otherwise. In 1991, one psychiatrist actually met the requirements for using hallucinogens in clinical research with humans. Psychiatrist and hallucinogen researcher Rick Strassman explained it this way: "The reflex reactions of interested parties are being replaced by more measured responses to issues regarding the study of these drugs."[103]

"TRAIN COMIN' THROUGH. RIGHT NOW."[104]

In 1990 Strassman was the first researcher since 1970 to get federal funding to study hallucinogens, specifically DMT, in human volunteers. At the time he was an associate professor in the Psychiatry Department at the University of New Mexico School of Medicine in Albuquerque. Why did he decide to study hallucinogens in people with a kick-butt drug that never

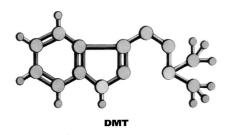

DMT

even made the *Lifetime Prevalence of the Use of Various Drugs in U.S. Households, Persons Aged 12 and Older, by Age Group, 1991*? DMT was a good candidate for reopening human research because it was well-characterized and had relatively typical (for hallucinogens) neuropharmacologic and behavioral properties. Its short-term action, relative obscurity and history of safe use in clinical research were a bonus. And something else made it interesting.

◤ INTERLUDE: YOUR BRAIN IS A DRUG LAB

Give me Librium® or give me meth.
—Mart Crowley, *The Boys in the Band*

**Benzodiazepines, Xanax® and gin
Somebody's feeling no pain...**
—Leo Kottke, "Big Mob on the Hill"
Great Big Boy, (Chrysalis Records)

DMT WAS DISCOVERED IN PLANTS, but researchers learned later that it was endogenous in lower animals and humans. Yes! They found it in human brain tissue—a mind-blowing hallucinogen. So, like any other drug, to work in the brain DMT had to bind to a receptor. Now researchers knew *why* the brain had DMT receptors—because

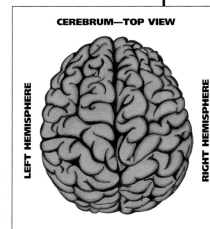

CEREBRUM—TOP VIEW

LEFT HEMISPHERE

RIGHT HEMISPHERE

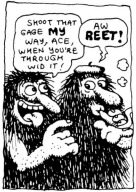

it had DMT (why it was there, what role it played, was a whole other question).

But the brain had receptors for opiates, too, like morphine and heroin; and benzodiazepines like Librium and Valium; and later even for delta-9-tetrahydrocannabinol (THC), the main psychoactive element in marijuana and hashish. Did that mean the brain made natural compounds just like morphine, Valium and THC?

THE BRAIN'S OWN BENZODIAZEPINES[105]

Researchers at the Roche Drug Co. in Nutley, New Jersey, developed the best-known benzodiazepines, Librium (1960) and Valium (1963). The new drugs relieved anxiety but didn't make users as sleepy as barbiturates like Seconal and Nembutal did, and they weren't as addicting. In 1977, independent research teams (at Roche in Basel and Ferrosan in Copenhagen) discovered receptors for Valium in rat neuron membranes. In 1978, a researcher at the National Institute of Mental Health (NIMH) discovered a relationship between Valium receptors and receptors for the inhibitory neurotransmitter GABA (gamma aminobutyric acid, the same receptors alcohol binds to).

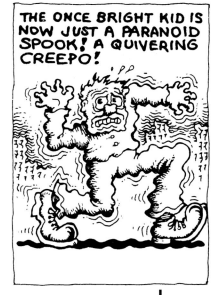

THE ONCE BRIGHT KID IS NOW JUST A PARANOID SPOOK! A QUIVERING CREEPO!

Later research showed that GABA and benzodiazepine receptors shared the same large protein molecule, and that benzodiazepines worked by boosting GABA's inhibitory effect on neurons in the brain. But they still didn't know why a GABA-benzodiazepine receptor evolved over millions of years in the first place. No, the Roche guys didn't travel back in time and plant a benzodiazepine receptor in some unsuspecting hominid.

Some scientists thought it meant the brain maybe had a natural chemical that's a lot like the benzodiazepines. No one's found anything yet, but that's okay. It took decades to find receptors for the endogenous opiates called endorphins (or enkephalines)—morphine-like compounds made in the brain.

Sol Snyder again: "It seems likely that the benzodiazepine receptor sites are part of a natural mechanism that normally regulates the kinds of emotional states" that get changed in people who have symptoms of anxiety.[106]

THE BRAIN'S OWN THC

IN 1988,[107] William Devane discovered that neuron membranes had protein receptors that bound THC. That a THC receptor exists in the brain implied the human brain made a compound just like THC. Scientists all over the world started looking for it. Meanwhile, Devane went to Hebrew University in Jerusalem to work with chemist Raphael Mechoulam, who'd first determined the structure of THC molecules. In 1992, Devane and colleagues found the compound in pig brains. They called it anandamide, from the Sanskrit word *ananda* meaning bliss. In 1993 Devane went to the National Institute of Mental Health in Bethesda, Maryland, to continue his work.

Back at Hebrew University, Mechoulam and his team identified two more fatty acid ethanolamides (like anandamide) that bind to the cannabinoid receptor. No one knows the biological role of anandamides yet, but Mechoulam thinks they might help coordinate movement and may be involved in biochemically turning objective reality into subjective emotions.

It *does* take people who witness a disaster a second or two to react—you can see that clearly in footage of the audience present at the January 1986 *Challenger* launch and explosion: people smiling and cheering. Cut to explosion. The people freeze in confusion. Seconds later the screaming starts.

Here's how it might work, using the 1995 bombing of the federal building in Oklahoma City as an example. The entire process takes seconds.

> Someone nearby **HEARS** the blast and **WATCHES** the huge federal building collapse into dust and debris.

This is straight video and audio input to the witness's brain. No emotions yet.

> **NOW QUESTIONS:** What was that? What could have blown? How many people are in there? Did it affect his [floor, division, mainframe, working group]?

If the role of anandamides in the brain is to biochemically turn objective reality into subjective emotions, this is where they might come in. Maybe the brain has

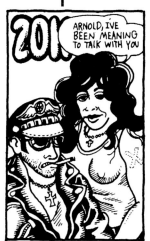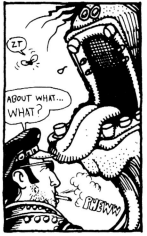

an anandamide system that handles, bit by bit, the whole incoming reality stream. It would monitor objective data bits for potential interest; trash most of them and mark the rest biochemically, according to a person's dynamic hot list of interests; then channel the high-priority stuff to Emotion Central and it all emerges as output in the form of laughing, screaming, crying, fainting, smirking or running. Or whatever.

TRIPS: HOW HALLUCINOGENS WORK IN YOUR BRAIN

THE EMOTIONS HE FEELS depend on who he is—the husband or father of someone in the building (horror, grief), a worker returning late from a coffee break (shock, relief) or the bomber (excitement, fear).

1990-1991: BACK TO DMT

Starting in 1991, Rick Strassman and colleagues at the University of New Mexico's General Clinical Research Center studied DMT's effects in 12 volunteers who were experienced hallucinogen users. The following report is from his research summary.

Strassman's approach was to study volunteers who'd already used lots of different hallucinogens. His group believed only experienced users could deal with possible bad reactions to DMT—a 30-minute, highly disruptive drug the volunteers would take while wired to medical monitoring equipment in the gleaming sterility of a clinical research center. To quantify DMT effects, the team developed the Hallucinogen Rating Scale (see "Other Stuff" at the back of the book) based on descriptions from users of DMT and other hallucinogens.

Volunteers got several different doses of DMT, but this summary only covers those who got 0.4 mg/kg intravenously, the highest hallucinogenic dose. They were almost uniformly overwhelmed at the effects and how fast they came on. Even before they got the full dose, volunteers described an intense, usually temporary, anxiety-causing rush through their bodies and minds. Some compared it with a freight train—it immediately replaced normal mental function with hallucinogenic effects. Some volunteers forgot they had bodies and, for the first minute or two, many forgot they were in a hospital as part of a research project.

Visual imagery was the most noticeable effect. At this dose they saw images with their eyes opened or closed. The images were familiar and novel—a fantastic bird, a tree of life and knowledge, a ballroom with crystal chandeliers, humans and aliens, a computer motherboard, ducts, DNA double helices, a pulsating diaphragm, a spinning golden disk, a huge fly eye bouncing in front of someone's face, tunnels and stairways.

Further into the drug trial, some volunteers opened their eyes and said the visual field was undulating and overlaid with geometric patterns; colors were more intense. Several described a visual-perceptual continuity problem that interfered with their normal ability to process what they saw. Most subjects said the room was much more than three-dimensional.

During the initial drug rush, nearly half the volunteers heard sounds that were high-pitched, whining/whirring, chattering, crinkling/crunching or comical, like 'boing-sproing' cartoon sounds. Body effects were like a stimulatory fear response, then progressed to a sense of detachment or dissociation from the body. Losing awareness of physical experience coincided with the most intense display of hallucinatory images.

Some male subjects described a sexual effect—a hot, pleasurable sensation in the genital area. No one had an orgasm or ejaculated. Some described a sense of flying or falling or a sense of decreased body weight or rapid movement. Sensations of hot, warm and cold were common. The volunteers were

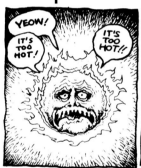 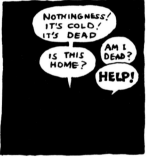

anxious as the rush developed, but they settled into the experience 15 to 30 seconds after the injection. More experienced users could disassociate emotional responses from the physical fear response. Most described the high dose as exciting, euphoric and positively charged, associating feelings with the visual display. It wasn't unusual for a volunteer to have very different emotional reactions that alternated or existed simultaneously—like fear and euphoria, anxiety and relaxation.

Volunteers found the high dose compelling, novel, unusual and a little disorienting. But after some initial confusion they maintained a watchful, observing ego. They almost uniformly said their thinking processes were qualitatively unchanged, and many said the processes sped up. The volunteers' reality testing was affected when they were so absorbed in the DMT effects that they forgot they were in an experimental setting. Others compared their experiences at this dose with dreams. Some volunteers came out of the experience with new perspectives on their personal or professional lives.

The first high dose usually made people more anxious, especially the first 30 seconds after injection, than a later high dose. Volunteers were ready to lose control after the first experience. But they understood the drug experi-

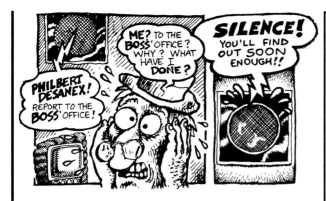

ence was essentially safe and that they wouldn't die or lose their minds, so were strengthened by the first high dose. And they were confident the research team would support their regressed states as the study progressed.

◣ RICK STRASSMAN SEZ

"Our first DMT study was a dose-response study. It was descriptive as opposed to trying to tease apart which receptors mediated which specific effects. But before you start pharmacologically dissecting the effects you see with the drug, you have to carefully characterize the effects—as endocrine, behavioral, cardiovascular and other autonomic effects. Once we characterized DMT's effects in our group, we could start designing more experimental studies. I finished one study that attempted to block the 5-HT$_{1A}$ receptor. All the tryptamines, DMT in particular, have a high affinity for the 5-HT$_{1A}$ subtype. I blocked it with a drug called pindolol. We had volunteers come in four times and each time gave them a different drug combination—the classic four-cell design when you deal with two drugs at once. One combination was DMT and pindolol, one was DMT and placebo pindolol, one was pindolol and placebo DMT, and one was placebo DMT and placebo pindolol.

"We essentially compared people's psychological and biological responses to DMT alone with their

TRIPS: LONG & SHORT

☛Intravenous DMT is an ultrashort-acting drug. It comes on in less than a minute, peaks within five minutes, and is over in less than 30 minutes.

☛Intramuscular DMT is a short-acting drug. It comes on in minutes, peaks in 15 minutes, ends in about an hour.

☛Intermediate-acting hallucinogens include the orally active psilocybin. They come on in 15-30 minutes, peak at 1-3 hours, last up to 6 hours.

☛Long-acting hallucinogens are LSD and mescaline. They come on in 30 to 90 minutes, peak at 3-5 hours, last 8-12 hours. Ultra long-acting compounds include ibogaine, the African plant that lasts 18-24 hours.

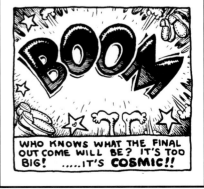

responses to DMT after their 5-HT$_{1A}$ receptors were blocked with pindolol. We found the psychological effects increased when we blocked the 5-HT$_{1A}$ site with pindolol. Our conclusion is that tryptamines activate the 5-HT$_{1A}$ and 5-HT$_2$ sites, and that stimulating the 5-HT$_{1A}$ site acts to buffer the effect of unrestrained 5HT$_2$ activation. Because 5-HT$_{1A}$ is an inhibitory receptor, if a couple of receptors mediate the same response and you block the one that's inhibitory, it's like taking the brakes off a response. Unopposed activation of the site could then be stronger.

"We found increased psychological responses to DMT with pindolol blockage. We also saw increased blood pressure responses to the combination compared with DMT itself. We found no change in a hormone called ACTH that rises with DMT, but we did find a reduced prolactin response to DMT when we combined it with pindolol. Our interpretation is that the 5-HT$_{1A}$ and 5-HT$_2$ sites both mediate DMT's effects.

"In terms of blood pressure and psychological responses, the 5-HT$_{1A}$ site is inhibitory. When you block it with pindolol, unopposed type 2 activity is unrestrained. In terms of the prolactin response, we hypothesized that the effect seen with DMT is more importantly mediated by the 5-HT$_{1A}$ site. Prolactin is a pituitary hormone responsible for milk production in women after childbirth, and involved with mood in women and men. An important aspect of the pindolol results is that one receptor type mediates some DMT effects, and another receptor type mediates others.

"It's quite interesting to have one drug that affects multiple sites in the brain. You can tease them apart to see which receptor mediates which drug effects. The important quality of these drugs is the psychological effects they engender. The only way to determine psychological effects and the effect of manipulating the pharmacology on the responses to psychedelics is to study a human being who experiences the psychological effects and can report on them.

"The thing that's so interesting about the state of the art of human psychedelic research is that these compounds have been well studied in lower animals in the laboratory for the last 20 or 25 years. We have a huge amount of preclinical data from lower animals that point to the human experiments that should be done now.

"If we understand what receptor in lower animals mediates either electrophysiological or behavioral changes, and if somebody's interested in blocking the effects of LSD in an emergency room on someone having a bad trip, one's choice of drugs to block the effects in a person would be informed by the human research that would have taken place based on research findings in lower animals.

"I believe that fundamentally our knowledge of animal pharmacology of hallucinogen effects is adequate. Not that we don't need new drugs or that the understanding of hallucinogens is complete. But an enormous amount of work on hallucinogens is waiting to be done in humans solely from a psychological perspective. Because the psychology and inner worlds of animals are so different from ours, we ought to pay more attention to characterizing the psychological effects of these drugs in humans.

"For example, how important are set and setting in hallucinogen responses? Who might benefit from hallucinogen-assisted psychotherapy? What are the characteristics of effective hallucinogen-assisted psychotherapy practitioners? While pharmacology may underpin all this, the real bread-and-butter data are human, subjective and interpersonal.

"Most people who want to be able to prescribe and give and take these drugs are not only concerned with reversing disordered brain metabolism. They're into depressed people feeling better, creative people being more creative, confused people being less confused—all human mental problems. I don't think it makes sense to approach it purely biologically while relegating subjective experience to a lesser role; the inner experience is so important.

"People are a rich source of data, my questionnaire is based on what somebody says, what they see and feel, their thinking and perception. The rating scale results were more sensitive than any biological data in our studies. I think that's important."

1992: AN UPDATE ON HALLUCINOGENS

In 1992, NIDA sponsored a two-day technical meeting for hallucinogen researchers in Bethesda, Maryland, called *Hallucinogens: An Update*. Rick Strassman was the only one there who had federal authorization *and* funding to study psychedelics in human volunteers.

But the other 20 or so researchers were doing important work—the kind that didn't exist in the '60s because the technology didn't exist: molecular studies of LSD, DMT, mescaline and their sites of action in the brain; and MRI and PET scans that showed where hallucinogens went in the brain to put on their show.

Also in 1992, NIDA assembled leading researchers to discuss the status of research on LSD and similar drugs, and to decide whether hallucinogens were potentially therapeutic and how best to study them. At the meeting, researchers said they needed new human hallucinogen data, not more animal studies. Soon after, NIDA presented its technical-review results to the FDA's

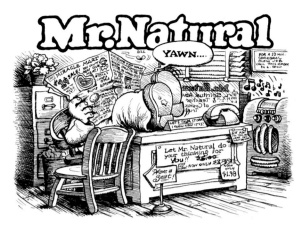

Drug Abuse Advisory Committee, which met to reconsider human clinical investigations and investigational new drug studies on hallucinogens. The committee decided to evaluate hallucinogen applications case by case, and approve them if they met the same rigorous standards FDA required for investigating any new drug.[108]

 1993: 50 YEARS OF LSD

During the last week of October 1993, the Swiss Academy of Medical Sciences held a meeting in Lugano-Agno, a city in Switzerland surrounded by mountain lakes and so close to Italy's border that everyone spoke Italian. Researchers streamed in from all over the globe to attend what may have been one of the planet's most esoteric conferences —*50 Years of LSD: Current Status and Perspectives of Hallucinogens.*

LSD-developer Albert Hofmann was star of the show and after-dinner speaker. He was in his eighties. This was the chemist who had made it all possible—Haight-Ashbury, Timothy Leary, the Summer of Love, long hair, free love, changed minds, socio-intellectual pharmacological rebellion, hip-

50 YEARS OF LSD
STATE OF THE ART AND
PERSPECTIVES OF HALLUCINOGENS

SYMPOSIUM
OF THE SWISS ACADEMY OF MEDICAL SCIENCES
OCTOBER 21 AND 22, 1993
LUGANO-AGNO (SWITZERLAND)

pies, acid rock and indirectly, god help him, bell bottoms—by discovering "the fantastic effects of LSD on the human psyche" on April 19, 1943, in his lab at Sandoz.[109]

The meeting at Lugano-Agno was the first of its kind in decades because long hair and acid rock weren't the only mutations that seeped into the mainstream from the 1960s counterculture. Taboos that sprung from the barrage of '60s drug misinformation were still very big, especially those involving hallucinogens and humans. It had been a long time since anyone in the U.S. except Rick Strassman had studied hallucinogens in people. But by 1992, most investigators knew about Strassman's approved protocol and his National Institute on Drug Abuse (NIDA) funding for DMT studies with human volunteers.

The field looked like it might be moving again, and the 50th anniversary LSD meeting attracted researchers and government regulators from Germany, Switzerland, France, the United Kingdom and the United States.

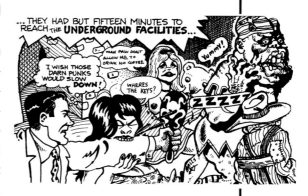

It was weird but fascinating, a reunion of scientists, former colleagues, co-workers and collaborators who traded esoteric but apparently side-splitting technical anecdotes, professional gossip, research plans, business cards, bureaucratic horror stories and e-mail addresses. Each attendee got an armload of stuff—Swiss cookies; a ceramic mug handmade in Basel, where Hofmann developed LSD-25; and a personalized Swiss Academy of Medical Sciences rubber briefcase with Sandoz-imprinted paper, pencils and pens. Sandoz was a corporate sponsor even though it hadn't marketed LSD since 1966.

As the meeting opened, symposium chairman Alfred Pletscher took the microphone and addressed a full house. Maybe 125 people, among them some of the world's premier hallucinogen researchers, many in their sixties, seventies and eighties.

"How many in the room have taken LSD?" Pletscher wanted to know. "Will you raise your hands?" 75 or 80 hands went up. Every neck in the place swiveled. It was probably the only place on earth where so many of the raised hands clutched Sandoz pens and belonged to grinning, tweedy, bespectacled guys with white hair. At the

ALFRED PLETSCHER

50th anniversary of LSD's discovery in Switzerland, with Albert Hofmann in the room, it was a peak experience.

On the second day of the meeting, Dr. Geraline Lin rose from the audience and said a few words about federal attitudes toward hallucinogens. She's a program officer from the Basic Research Division at NIDA, a main

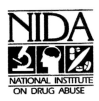

NATIONAL INSTITUTE
ON DRUG ABUSE

source of federal funding for hallucinogen research in the United States.

"It's a good sign," she said, "that a little over a year ago NIDA revived its interest in hallucinogens. We feel we should give this type of drug a fair chance for investigation—a chance to undergo the same stringent, vigorous, scientifically sound, well-controlled and [well-]designed study as other classes of drugs. NIDA is oriented to preventing drug abuse, but we're also interested in the process of doing so because of LSD's profound actions on consciousness and its immense impact on individual and public health. We hope, by subjecting this class of drugs to vigorous investigation, to either account for or discount undesirable effects and potential therapeutic utility, if any. That would be a great service to the scientific community and to public health.

"We're interested in developing a study design for clinical trials. We're working closely with the FDA on a protocol [standard procedure] for studying hallucinogenic drugs, and we work closely with DEA, a federal agency with drug control and scheduling authority, and FDA, which is responsible for approving investigational new drug applications. Investigators have to go over a lot of hurdles to do research in this area.

"By developing this sound protocol with hallucinogen researchers and regulatory and drug enforcement agencies, we hope to open the door for clinical hallucinogen research and gain insight into the mechanisms of action of these drugs. And we hope that, 50 years from now, we'll have the solid scientific base we need to clarify, justify or discount some claims commonly attributed to hallucinogen use. We also hope to be able to put hallucinogens in their rightful place in the scientific arena, without having to apologize because they weren't subject to stringent scientific scrutiny."

As the meeting closed another speaker, Dieter Ladewig, wrapped up. He's an associate professor of psychiatry and head of the Addiction & Alcoholism Treatment and Research Unit in the University of Basel Psychiatry Department. In the last 50 years, he said, researchers had learned a lot about LSD's mechanisms of action. But they still hadn't settled the debate on whether hallucinogens were clinically useful—for treating neuroses, autism, schizophrenia, alcoholism and as a therapeutic element for terminal patients. The challenge is to integrate animal and human research to answer questions

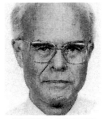

DIETER LADEWIG

like—Why do hallucinogens affect different people in different ways? What's the basis of vulnerability to problems with hallucinogens? Which patients can be treated with hallucinogens, in which therapeutic settings, with which drugs?

The therapeutic use of hallucinogens must be reevaluated, Ladewig concluded. Swiss authorities had been open-minded about hallucinogen therapy, but health authorities in the United States, the United Kingdom, Germany and elsewhere should reconsider their moratorium on human clinical research and let investigators study the psychopharmacology of hallucinogens in people.[110]

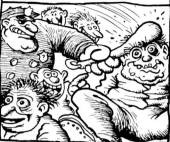

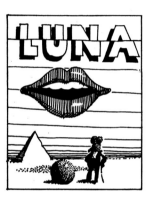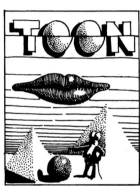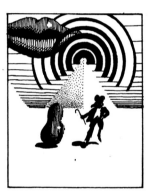

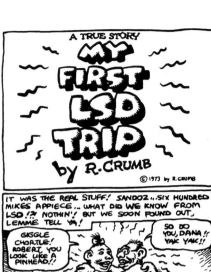

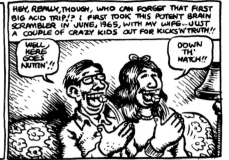

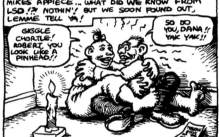

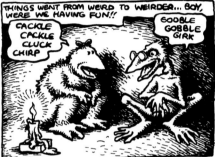

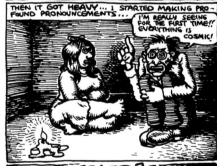

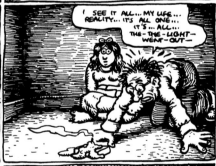

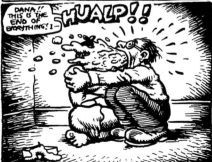

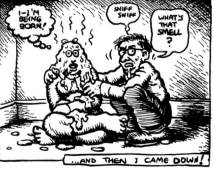

PART III

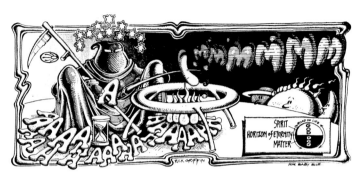

Chapter 8

L S D :   H E R E   N O W

LSD IS THE WORLD'S most notorious hallucinogen, but way too many people, including some with medical degrees and some who've used LSD for years, can't describe its basic characteristics. LSD ultimately is derived from ergot, a fungus that grows on rye and other grains. It's been around since the 1940s. Caffeine and aspirin break chromosomes but LSD doesn't. And there's no such thing as the kind of cheesy LSD flashbacks they used to 'simulate' with weird music and out-of-focus camera lenses on *Mod Squad*. Technically, LSD users don't even hallucinate. People who have true hallucinations—like schizophrenics—believe what they see is real. People who drop 200+ micrograms (mcg) of LSD are blown away by what they see and hear but know exactly why it's happening and remember it later—after the buildings stop melting into the ground. Early LSD

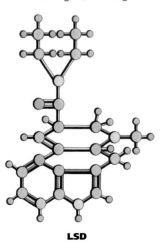

LSD

research showed a clinical pattern of vivid perceptual distortions, not the true hallucinations associated with schizophrenia. But it's still really hard to drive. And forget juggling.

Hallucinogens are different from other psychoactive drugs (like booze, speed or downers) that cause perceptual distortions, delusions and other changes in thinking, behavior and mood—and LSD is considered the proto-typical psychedelic compound. People who take psychedelics can experience states of altered perception, thought and feeling that usually only happen in dreams or spiritual states. LSD generates physical and mental effects that vary among people who take it according to their personality and—at the time—mood, expectations, setting and dose. DEA and lots of other sources say typ-

HALLUCINOGENS & CHEMICAL FAMILIES
Phenethylamines mescaline
Indolealkylamines psilocybin, DMT
Lysergamides LSD, morning glory seeds

ical LSD doses in the 1990s range from 20 to 80 mcg. In the 1960s and early '70s, doses were more like 250+ mcg. Just as a personal observation, this is roughly the difference between feeling mildly euphoric during a con-cert (20-80 mcg), not being able to tell—except by closely studying people around you—which way to turn to face the band (150-275 mcg), whatever *that* is (300-450+ mcg).

PEOPLE WHO TAKE oral LSD can have dilated pupils, nausea, flushing, chills, higher blood pressure and heart rate, tremor, weakness and dizziness. Psychological effects within 30-90 minutes could include inner tension; fast chang-ing moods; visual, auditory and sensory illusions and distortions; synesthesia (hearing sights, see-ing sounds); a sense that time is running slow; ego dissolution, detachment or fragmentation; recalling old memories; and a sense that every-thing's meaningful. Everyone who takes high-dose LSD has sensory-cue slip-ups: after-images

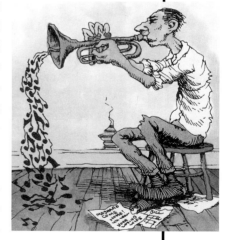

last a long time and leave trails, flat surfaces look deep, inanimate things (walls, paintings) seem to breathe. And it's impossible to predict behavior because individual reactions to LSD depend on dose, setting, expectations, personality and emotional stress.

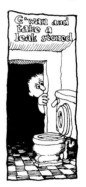

Albert Hofmann described his own LSD experience pretty well in *LSD: My Problem Child*, and you could raise the global temperature 1 degree by burning all the tedious descriptions in books and on the Net of personal hallucinogen experiences. But basically, at doses above about 200 mcg, there's no such thing as a straight line; whatever you look at breathes, changes color faster than Dennis Rodman's hair, and morphs continually into and out of (what looks like) animation. For the closest thing to hallucinogenic visual distortions, see the 'Toon Town sequence in *Who Framed Roger Rabbit?*,* when Bob Hoskins drives out of a tunnel and into... heaving landscapes! cackling trees! cars with faces! And buildings that sway and melt into the whole chaotic color bleed.

Everything not heaving or churning has some kind of undulating geometric pattern all over it, including the air. Your sense of time and space goes in the (cosmic) toilet. Some people have religious or mystical experiences. LSD lasts 9-12 hours. As it wears off, people who've had a good experience are calm, energetic and have a sense of detachment and control. If the LSD experience wasn't positive, well... That's another story, isn't it?[111]

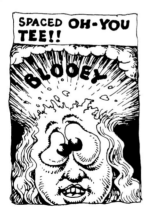

WHAT A BUMMER

In 1984, psychiatrist Rick Strassman surveyed the literature on bad trips in "Adverse Reactions to Psychedelic Drugs: A Review of the Literature." The problem with those studies is that the researchers usually had no information about patients' medical and psychiatric histories. Here's an edited version of his summary and conclusions:

From the mid-1950s to mid-1960s, psychiatrists and psychotherapists had a great burst of enthusiasm for the therapeutic, growth-enhancing value of LSD and other psychedelics. In the mid-to-late '60s, a growing number of reports of adverse and occasionally lethal reactions to psychedelics (and god knows *what* else)

---

*Steven Spielberg & Robert Zemeckis, *Who Framed Roger Rabbit?*, Touchstone Pictures, 1988. "The chemistry," says a review on the home video cover, "is magic..."

taken on the street made it hard for legitimate researchers to get and study psychedelics in humans. But the black market never closes, and in the 1980s it was the sole producer of current data on human hallucinogen use. Its sub-

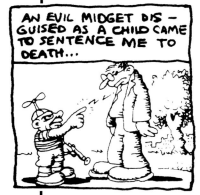

jects were the street-drug-using "LSD casualties" who shuffled around at major psychiatric research centers. The most common adverse reaction was a panic episode—a bad trip—that lasted less than 24 hours. Symptoms included scary visual and auditory illusions or hallucinations, anxiety to the point of panic, aggression, depression, confusion and fear to the point of paranoid delusions. Reactions that lasted days or months or sent people to the hospital were LSD psychoses. These happened most often to people who had problems before they took LSD or who had histories of psychiatric treatment or drug use. But good reactions and bad reactions can happen to anyone, any time.

According to the literature, the rate of bad trips was low when normal volunteers and patients were carefully screened, prepared, supervised, followed up, and given reasonable doses of a pharmaceutical-quality drug. The few *prospective** studies that mentioned bad reactions consistently described patients whose psychiatric profiles or histories of drug use predicted a poor response to psychedelics. But most studies of multiple bad trips were *retrospective*** and described similar characteristics in street-drug users who sought treatment for bad trips. In studies that discussed the relationship between drug-induced mental illness and mentally ill people who

*In research, a *prospective* study is one where the investigators use their own protocol and research subjects [people, animals, whatever] and report the results they get from that group.

**In a *retrospective* study, researchers get their results by using data from earlier studies by other investigators.

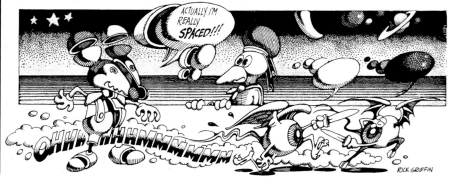

A SUMMARY OF LSD USE

from *LSD: Still With Us After All These Years* by Leigh A. Henderson and William J. Glass (New York: Lexington Books, 1994): 97-98.

The main concerns about LSD are that more school-age kids are using it and that they're younger than past users. Drug-use data doesn't support either concern. But it does show that, after intense interest and experimentation in the late 1960s and early 1970s, LSD use settled into a pattern in a limited population. In some ways it looks like a disease that constantly circulates at low levels in a population.

LSD use was fairly steady between the late 1970s and early 1990s. The media periodically report local LSD outbreaks, but there's not much evidence for a nationwide epidemic. Some U.S. communities report increasing LSD use; others report none. Regional fluctuations in LSD supply and demand seem to be part of its pattern. No one's reported any recent large national increases in LSD supplies.

National surveys suggest that most LSD users are white, male and middle-to-upper class. Their interest in trying LSD peaks in late adolescence. They've probably used alcohol, marijuana and maybe inhalants and over-the-counter drugs; they'll probably use LSD a few times.

The average user tries LSD at 17, so half of those who use LSD do it before they're 17. LSD use for 9-year-olds has been consistently reported over 15 to 20 years, but actual use at this age is low and the data doesn't show it increasing. Most high school students who report using LSD try it once or twice. Even among the small number who use it more often, most stop by their early 20s. Only a small portion use LSD into their 30s. LSD rarely causes reactions that need emergency medical care. When it does happen, other drugs are also usually involved, and patients are treated and released.

LSD is one of many drugs adolescents are exposed to; those who use LSD probably will already have tried (and may still use) other drugs. High school students use LSD less often than they use alcohol, marijuana, cocaine or over-the-counter or prescription drugs. Younger students inhale potentially lethal substances like solvents and butane more often than they use LSD.

used psychedelics, most focused on schizophrenia-like illnesses and showed a similar clinical picture and course for (hallucinogen-using or not) schizophrenics. Some mentioned a possible relationship between mood disorders and LSD psychosis. Researchers had studied long-term LSD effects in different settings and populations. In normal volunteers, objective data didn't seem to tap the subjective sense of peoples' changed internal worlds, but people who used LSD regularly to alter consciousness showed personality and coping styles. In the few large caseload reports on long-term psychiatric effects of LSD, the very tentative conclusion was that in fringe-element people chronic, heavy LSD use seemed to produce a disorder that resists treatment. (This is bad news, but not for the people taking LSD. Ego syntonic means 'relatively agreeable to the person in question.' And it resists treatment. What—they can't get the chronic, fringe-element LSD users to stop smiling? For the drug-use-equals-drug-abuse crowd, it sorta sucks the symmetry out of their lethal LSD effects list— PSYCHOSIS! INSANITY!

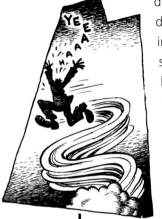

SUICIDE! *AND* AN AGREEABLE MENTAL STATE THAT DOESN'T GO AWAY FOR A *REAL LONG TIME!*) But comprehensive, well-controlled studies of neuropsychological function showed no big differences between groups of LSD users and non-users.

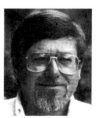

ADOLF DITTRICH

➤ LSD & ALTERED STATES[112]

In 1985, Adolf Dittrich and a big research team published the results of an International Study on Altered States of Consciousness. The study involved

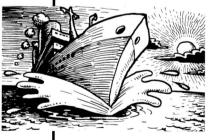

1,133 people from seven countries—Switzerland, Germany, Great Britain, Italy, Switzerland, Portugal and the United States. Their results showed that the basic dimensions of an LSD experience are a lot like experiences that come from other hallucinogens or from non-drug experiences like sensory deprivation or some kinds of sensory overload. Their conclusion—basically that altered states of consciousness from LSD, DMT or hypnosis are pretty much the same, psychologically.

In an article on the psychological aspects of LSD-based altered states, Dittrich defined an *altered state of consciousness* as a change in thinking—a changed sense of time; a feeling of lost control; intense emotions; a changed body image; a change in visual perception including pseudo-hallucinations, visions, illusions or synesthesia; and a change in the meanings of some beliefs. All this stuff fits into three categories of feelings that Dittrich says make up the altered state—oceanic boundlessness, a state like a mystical experience; fear of ego dissolution, an unpleasant state similar to what people call a bad trip; and visual restructuralization, which includes pseudo-hallucinations or visions, illusions and synesthesia.

People who tend to experience oceanic boundlessness during altered states are usually extroverts and optimistic toward life. Altered states usually:

 Represent a big change in subjective experience or psychological function of normal people from normal waking consciousness. Mood and motor activity can change, and people can have unusual experiences of themselves and their environment—like separate realities in time and space.

 Last only a few hours, compared with psychiatric disorders that can last years or a lifetime.

 Are induced voluntarily or happen spontaneously; are not the result of illness or adverse circumstances.

 Are considered irrational, abnormal, exotic or pathological compared with the social norms of mainstream society.

DAVID NICHOLS SEZ

DAVID NICHOLS

From a June 1996 telephone interview with David Nichols, Ph.D., professor of medicinal chemistry and pharmacology, Department of Medicinal Chemistry and Molecular Pharmacology at Purdue University, West Lafayette, Indiana.

"At its heart, medicinal chemistry really is a study of the relationship between a chemical molecule and its biological activity. What are the relationships between the structural chemical features of a drug molecule and its biological effects? That can involve drug design or analysis of drug action or synthesis of drugs with the idea of modifying different parts of the molecules so you look at the consequences on biological activity.

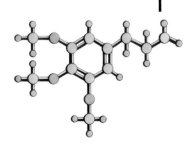

MESCALINE

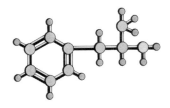

AMPHETAMINE

"With the hallucinogens we know a lot more now than we used to, but there's still plenty to understand. We know pretty precisely what the optimal structural features are in certain types of psychedelic classes. In mescaline analogs and amphetamines, for example, if you distill the work we've done and that [chemist Alexander] Shulgin and [medicinal chemist Richard] Glennon have done, you can say—Okay, if you have a benzene ring attached to two carbons attached to a nitrogen, which has two hydrogens on it and you have a methoxy at the 2 position and a methoxy at the 5 position and some large hydrophobic group at the 4 position, this is as good as it gets in terms of potency.

"With the LSD molecule, we know quite a bit about that structure. Same thing with the psilocybin/psilocin-type compounds; we can pretty precisely define the recognition aspects of the molecules that lead to highest activity. Now we're trying to connect that with elements in the receptor we think bind to them so we can look at the complementarity [to find out] what in the receptor interacts with that group to produce a response. But we're still in the dark ages in terms of the [LSD] receptors and the brain area and all that. That's still voodoo. We know what the amino acid sequences are of most of the receptors we're interested in, and there's a template. We think they resemble a molecule known as rhodopsin [the pigment sensitive to light in the eye's retina]. We think receptors have the general shape rhodopsin has; it's huge and indecipherable.

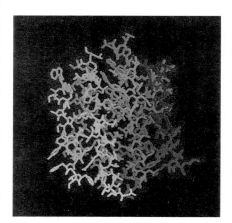
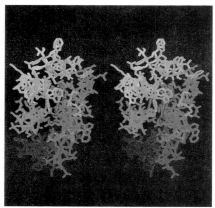

RHODOPSIN IMAGES: The large picture is an edge-on view of rhodopsin, missing its hydrogen atoms. Rhodopsin consists of 7 helices, each represented by a different color. The stereo view, according to Dr. David Nichols, "seems to be of the *crossed-eyes* variety. If you cross your eyes and look at it, then relax your eyes until you see three images and focus on the central image, it will be in stereo." Source: Brookhaven National Laboratory Protein Data Bank.

"[In terms of binding sites in the brain,] we haven't discovered any interactions besides the 5-HT$_{2A}$ and 5-HT$_{2C}$ receptors for amphetamine-type compounds like DOI, DOB or mescaline. Some new subtypes haven't been examined yet—like 5-HT$_6$ and 5-HT$_7$—and there may be other types we haven't found yet. If you look at rat or human data, there's a pretty direct correlation between potency in humans and the ability to activate the 5-HT$_{2A}$ receptor. The tryptamines [like DMT] are a little different because, in addition to the 5-HT$_{2A}$ and 5-HT$_{2C}$ effects, they have relatively high affinity for the 5-HT$_{1A}$ receptor, and this is also true for LSD.

"We don't know a lot about the 5-HT$_{1A}$ receptor but drug companies are interested in it because it may be involved in anxiety. One anti-anxiety drug—buspirone, sold as BuSpar—works by interacting with the 5-HT$_{1A}$ receptor in the brain stem and hippocampus. The mechanism of stimulating 5-HT$_{1A}$ receptors doesn't involve a neurochemical pathway that produces reinforcing effects, and there's interest because of the potential financial rewards of a nonaddictive anti-anxiety drug.

"I believe the 5-HT$_{1A}$ receptor is important to the actions of the tryptamines and LSD but I don't know exactly how it fits in. LSD also interacts with dopamine D$_1$ and D$_2$ receptors, serotonin receptors and others. So its effects go beyond the simple tryptamines and I suspect some affect the qualitative aspect of the [psychedelic experience]. Like a bottle of cheap red wine versus a bottle of fine, aged red wine that comes from a French vineyard and costs $180 a bottle. One has subtle nuances and bouquet [and the other doesn't].

"It would be a really long-term project with LSD to try to tease all that apart, but I think LSD is as potent as it is and as profound as it is to some extent because of the auxiliary things that happen beyond the central effects at 5-HT$_{2A}$, 5-HT$_{2C}$ and probably 5-HT$_{1A}$ receptors. Dopamine receptors are involved in the actions of things like psychostimulants—amphetamines, methamphetamine, cocaine. Most of those drugs produce euphoria. It may be that whatever euphoria LSD produces is partially related to its ability to interact with D$_1$ and D$_2$ receptors.

"[Drugs like MDA, MDMA and MDE] fall into some other category, some other class. They're not psychostimulants and they're not hallucinogens. We spent a

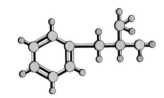

AMPHETAMINE

PSILOCYBIN

MDMA

long time trying to come up with a name for these drugs. Entactogen has Latin and Greek roots. *En* means 'inside,' *gen* means 'producing,' and *tactile* is from the Latin root *tactus*—touching. Tact also implies sensitivity and caring. These are drugs that produce a touching inside, and we wanted a name that set them apart from stimulants and hallucinogens. They give you access to things hidden inside by repressed memories. Psychiatrists think MDMA somehow releases repressed memories held in by emotional pain."

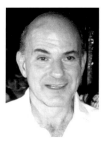

LSD & SEROTONIN

"From the very beginning, working with LSD turned out to be a literally maddening experience for many of us," George Aghajanian of Yale Medical School addressed members of the Serotonin Club at the Neuroscience Society's 25th annual meeting in 1995. "LSD has its good points. It got people interested in the field. It pointed out serotonin's possible significance because LSD was so potent it captured people's imaginations.

"But its bad points were a nightmare, especially in the dark years—the 1960s and earlier—before molecular biology was a standard research tool. LSD was incredibly complex, what pharmacologists call a dirty drug, because LSD seemed to work anywhere, at any receptor. No one could tell what was going on.

"So is that really the kind of drug one would want to work with?" Aghajanian shrugs. "At the time we didn't know better."

In the 1960s, some hallucinogen researchers suspected LSD might work through the brain's serotonin system. They didn't know the mechanism or whether other systems were involved, but they had tempting clues based mostly on parallels

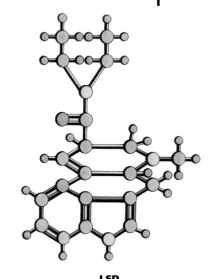

LSD

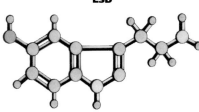

SEROTONIN (5-HT)

between LSD's effects and serotonin's chemical structure. No serotonin receptors were characterized at the time. Now, more than a dozen serotonin [receptors] are known and characterized, and hallucinogens act primarily on the 5-HT$_2$ class of receptors.

From a July 1996 telephone interview with George Aghajanian, M.D., Ph.D., an electrophysiologist and neuropharmacologist at the Yale University School of Medicine, and a long-time hallucinogen researcher.

"Our most recent work concentrates on 5-HT$_{2A}$ receptor function in the cerebral cortex, particularly the neocortex. That's where most of the receptors are and that's quite a logical place in thinking about what the hallucinogens do because they affect so many different kinds of function-cognition, mood, perception. The neocortex interprets incoming sensory information, it integrates sensory information with preexisting associations and controls motor output. All of those things get distorted [when people take LSD]... and the neocortex is where the 5-HT$_{2A}$ receptors are most concentrated. The 5-HT$_{2A}$ receptor is distributed in a very specific way throughout the entire neocortex, so it influences all cortical functions. The 5-HT$_{2C}$ receptor is not heavily represented in the neocortex, but it's in some other areas—the pyriform cortex and amygdala—so the 5-HT$_{2C}$ receptor is also a target for the hallucinogens. In animal studies the 5-HT$_{2C}$ receptor has been associated with anxiogenic [anxiety-producing] effects.

"I thought that possibly could explain [the fact that] there's often anxiety associated with the hallucinogens, and the 5-HT$_{2C}$ receptor might contribute to that. No one's actually doing the research yet, that I know of. [Blocking anxiety effects and leaving the purely psychedelic effects] is a theoretical possibility, and you probably couldn't get a good handle on that from the animal studies. It would be hard to know exactly how to compare the animal behavioral tests and the different human experiences.

"On a practical level, one way of putting the work on LSD and serotonin into perspective is this: the functions affected by messing around with 5-HT$_{2A}$ receptors, like the hallucinogens do, may be some of the same

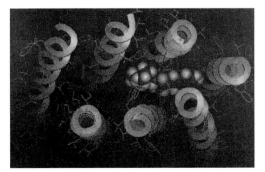

LSD BOUND TO THE 5-HT$_{2A}$ RECEPTOR: This is a representation of the LSD molecule docked inside the proposed ligand recognition site of the human serotonin 5-HT$_{2A}$ receptor, which is one member of the large family of G-protein coupled receptors. Source: Dr. David Nichols, president, the Heffter Research Institute. Used with permission.

functions that are disturbed in schizophrenia and other naturally occurring psychoses. Some of the newer, so-called atypical antipsychotic drugs, including clozapine and risperidone, are potent antagonists of the same receptor at which the hallucinogens are agonists. Hallucinogens stimulate the receptors and the new antipsychotic drugs block those receptors. Hallucinogens are partial agonists at 5-HT$_{2A}$ and 5-HT$_{2C}$ receptors. We don't fully understand [the significance of that] but we have some new ideas about it... like what 5-HT$_{2A}$ receptors actually do at the synaptic junction. In the neocortex they facilitate excitatory amino acid transmission (like that of glutamate, the brain's most common excitatory amino acid).

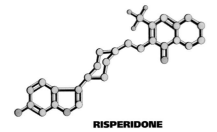

RISPERIDONE

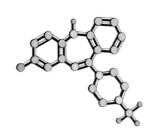

CLOZAPINE

"One of our ideas is that the natural transmitter has built into it actions at other serotonin receptors that counterbalance the increase in glutamatergic transmission, but the hallucinogens don't have that balanced effect so they facilitate glutamatergic transmission in an uncontrolled way [the neurons go wild]. That's one of the things we're playing around with now, but it's not far enough along to be more specific than that.

"[In terms of research progress on serotonin and LSD,] mechanistic human studies can now be done more intelligently because so much more is known about how the drugs work. We can now apply the mechanisms to human research, which wasn't possible 25 or 30 years ago because the 5-HT$_{2A}$ receptor wasn't even known then so there was no rationale for doing the studies. Years ago people were looking for hallucinogen antagonists as an antidote [to bad trips]. The other idea was finding a blocker for the hallucinogens would tell you something about how they worked. Now, all the evidence that the hallucinogens work through the 5-HT$_{2A}$ receptor and some specific 5-HT$_{2A}$-blocking drugs would allow one to approach the question in humans very specifically. That hasn't been done yet because of the problems in doing human research with [hallucinogens], but the new antipsychotic drugs should be excellent antidotes for LSD.

"From 1963 to 1965, while I was assigned to the Army Chemical Center at Edgewood Arsenal, I did some human studies and published a paper[113] on measuring blood levels of LSD in humans—the only study in existence like that. At that time there was an idea that maybe these drugs worked by triggering off

George Aghajanian explains
PARTIAL AGONISTS

"The maximum effect of a partial agonist like LSD, even if you use very high concentrations, is less than a substance like serotonin that's a full agonist. In systems where serotonin acts on 5-HT$_{2A}$ receptors, it has a certain maximum effect when you go up to the highest concentrations. Hallucinogens, even if you go to very high concentrations, only have 20 to 40 percent of the maximum effect of serotonin. They're partial in relation to serotonin. That's a very different concept from potency. If a compound is very potent, it means it does its thing at very low concentrations. Hallucinogens are much more potent than serotonin. There are scientists who don't even grasp that concept, and it's like the bread and butter of pharmacology.

"People tend to think something that's a partial agonist isn't very potent. But potency has nothing to do with the magnitude of the effect. Partial agonists can be twice as potent as a full agonist or very weak. The partial agonist idea has to do with the full magnitude of the effect. In pharmacology that concept is called efficacy—effectiveness. Let's say the maximum effect of serotonin at the 5-HT$_{2A}$ receptor is 10. At the same receptor, the maximum effect of LSD, no matter how high the concentration, is 2 or 3 of 10. That's what makes it a partial agonist. But LSD is still very powerful because it has its maximal effect at extremely low concentrations. With serotonin you need much higher concentrations to get a maximal effect. The fact that an effect is partial doesn't mean it isn't significant.

"Potency and efficacy—those are the two concepts. Efficacy has to do with the maximum effect; potency has to do with the amount you need to achieve the effect. Two drugs could have an identical effect, but you might have to use 100 pills of one and one pill of the other—that's very common. Another comparison is with mescaline and LSD. Mescaline is far less potent than LSD, so you have to use a lot more mescaline to get an effect than you have to do with LSD. But the effects are equivalent—they have similar efficacy. You can get just as good a hallucinogenic effect with mescaline as with LSD, but it takes a lot more mescaline. LSD is more potent than mescaline but it's no more efficacious."

SEROTONIN AS POLICE

from *Listening to Prozac* by Peter D. Kramer
(New York, Penguin Books, 1993): 327

No single theory covers the vast, complex body of work on depression at the level of the cell. Several inadequate models center on norepinephrine, and one very successful medication, Prozac, works through the serotonin system. One man who's worked for decades in this area has the following image of serotonin that guides his research: "Maybe serotonin is the police. The police aren't in one place... they cruise the city. Their potential presence makes you feel secure. If you don't have enough police, all sorts of things can happen. You may have riots. The absence of police doesn't cause riots. But if you have one and you don't have police, there's nothing to stop the riot from spreading." This doesn't explain everything that's known about the biochemistry of mood, but raising serotonin levels does seem to boost feelings of security, courage, assertiveness, self-worth, calm, flexibility and resilience. And serotonin-as-police addresses Prozac's usefulness in problems ranging from depression to obsessive-compulsive disorder. More generally, many things will go right when an animal, including a human animal, feels safe.

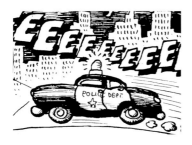

some event, then were rapidly cleared from the body. The hallucinogenic effects would persist in their own way and wouldn't need the presence of the drug. We showed that blood levels correlated highly with the psychological effects. That meant the drug effects depended on the drug occupying whatever receptor it was acting on.

"Knowing the [blood] levels of LSD in humans and the levels for LSD doses that produce psychological effects, we can get electrophysiological effects on neurons in rat brain slices that correspond to the levels we found in that early study. That tells us the effect we see at these low LSD concentrations are relevant to LSD effects in humans. In a recent article[114] we quoted the early study to show that LSD levels effective in our rat brain slices correspond to circulating levels of LSD in humans.

"There was a little controversy going on for a few years about whether hallucinogens are antagonists or agonists or partial agonists. So this [recent] study showed that in the pyriform cortex, hallucinogens are very potent partial agonists. Going back to the original context, LSD concentrations that were effective in the system were very similar to the circulating levels in humans we'd seen in the 1964 paper. [So at levels that are hallucinogenic in humans, DOI is a strong partial agonist.]"

"The only shared actions between the LSD-type and mescaline-type hallucinogens are at $5\text{-}HT_2$ receptors. That knowledge didn't exist in the '60s. $5\text{-}HT_2$ receptors weren't even proposed to exist until 1978, and they weren't cloned until more than 10 years later. The basic knowledge didn't exist in the '60s to figure out how hallucinogens worked. That's a huge difference between then and now. [Today] if someone has a bad trip, all the research findings say it should be possible to terminate the trip within half an hour using one of the newer antipsychotic drugs that blocks 5-HT$_2$ receptors.

"My own view of [the research] is that the hallucinogens tap into important mechanisms in the brain that involve a lot of other pathways. The importance of this research has to do with knowing more about those systems rather than the drugs per se. The ultimate interest is what it will tell us about the systems in the brain that are necessary to maintaining mental equilibrium."

And that's important, god knows.

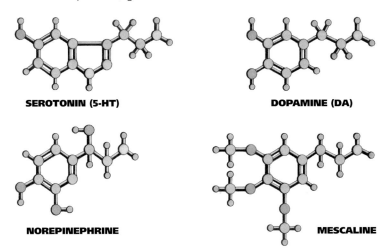

SEROTONIN (5-HT) DOPAMINE (DA)

NOREPINEPHRINE MESCALINE

SEROTONIN, HALLUCINOGENS & ANTIDEPRESSANTS

In the brain, most antidepressant drugs seem to work at serotonin, dopamine and norepinephrine receptors. Serotonin, dopamine and norepinephrine are also the main neurotransmitters [as far as anyone knows] involved in anxiety, depression *and* psychoactive drug effects.[115] That's no accident. Chemically, all the major psychedelics look so much like the neurotransmitters serotonin, dopamine or norepinephrine that they fit right into the same receptors. *That's* why hallucinogens work in your brain.

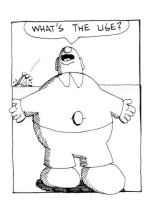

WHAT'S THE USE?

AFTER ANXIETY, depression's probably the most common mental problem on the planet. So the following information should be interesting to anyone who:

◎ has moods

◎ has a mood disorder

◎ uses hallucinogens

◎ has moods and uses hallucinogens

◎ has a mood disorder and uses hallucinogens.

DOCTORS WHO TREAT depressed patients probably tell them that some kinds of depression are caused by low levels or concentrations of serotonin in their brains, and they'll be taking a drug, probably a selective serotonin reuptake

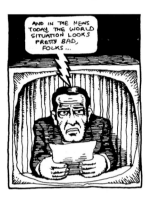

inhibitor (SSRI), to correct that. This is a great theory and lots of people use the model, but there's no hard evidence it's true. There's no test for living humans that directly measures serotonin concentrations in synapses between neurons in the brain. The only thing doctors can do, short of going in, is measure the amount of the serotonin metabolite, 5-hydroxyindole-acetic acid (5-HIAA) that accumulates in the spinal fluid. So if you haven't had a spinal tap lately, no one knows too much about your serotonin levels.

The most widely accepted hypothesis about depression involves biogenic amine neurotransmitter systems—like norepinephrine (called noradrenaline in Europe), serotonin and dopamine—that aren't working right. In this amine hypothesis, most forms of depression are brought on by low concentrations of norepinephrine, serotonin and maybe dopamine at important adrenergic (for norepinephrine), serotonergic (serotonin) and maybe dopaminergic (dopamine) receptors. So drugs that increase these concentrations at these receptors should reduce symptoms of depression.

To treat depression, doctors use stimulants that mimic norepinephrine, monoamine oxidase (MAO) inhibitors (tranylcypromine, phenelzine, isocarboxazid) that increase norepinephrine, serotonin and

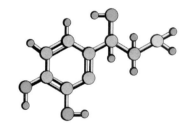

NOREPINEPHRINE (NE)

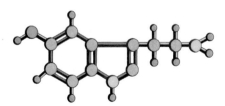

SEROTONIN (5-HT)

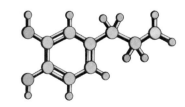

DOPAMINE (DA)

maybe dopamine concentrations by inhibiting their metabolism,[116] and tricyclic antidepressants (imipramine, desipramine, chlorpromazine) or selective

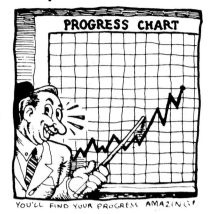

PROGRESS CHART

YOU'LL FIND YOUR PROGRESS AMAZING!

serotonin reuptake inhibitors—SSRIs like fluoxetine (Prozac), sertraline (Zoloft), paroxetine (Paxil)—that keep norepinephrine, serotonin and maybe dopamine loitering in the synapses after neurotransmission ends, and raise their concentrations in the brain. Prozac was the first of the new SSRIs and it's supposed to more specifically target serotonin and keep it active in certain brain systems with fewer side effects than older antidepressants.

Prozac and other SSRIs work mainly by blocking serotonin reuptake. This keeps serotonin from being sucked back up into the presynaptic neuron and recycled like old tires, and raises its concentrations around serotonin receptors in the brain. And, as one northern California researcher likes to say, "High-serotonin people are happy people." But that's just a theory.

Venlafaxine (Effexor), a newer antidepressant, chemically differs from tricyclics and SSRIs because it strongly inhibits serotonin and norepinephrine, and weakly inhibits dopamine uptake—so it raises levels of serotonin, norepinephrine and dopamine in the brain. It's as effective as tricyclics and, like SSRIs, has almost no side effects.

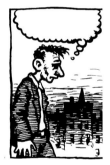

But don't forget: all doctors or pharmacologists really know is that when they give certain depressed people certain kinds of medications like Prozac (a few of them breathtakingly expensive), lots of depressive symptoms improve. That means the drugs can help treat some kinds of depression and suggests theories about why some people might get depressed. But right now there's no hard evidence to support the theories because of all the things no one knows for sure:

- The exact roles of serotonin, dopamine and norepinephrine in the brain
- How neurotransmitters work at their receptors
- What the receptors look like
- How and why antidepressants work
- Why some antidepressants work for some people and not for others
- What causes depression in the first place
- Why it takes some antidepressants 2-5 weeks to work.

AND THAT'S JUST FOR STARTERS. But given all the uncertainty, some of the theories hold up amazingly well.

IN 1994, PHARMACOLOGIST Katherine Bonson did a study at the National Institute of Mental Health (NIMH) on how hallucinogens and antidepressants interact in the brain. If you take antidepressants, psychedelics and recreational drugs, you'll want to put them all down for a minute and listen to this.

 KATHERINE BONSON SEZ

From an August 1996 telephone interview with pharmacologist Katherine Bonson, Ph.D., at NIMH, Bethesda, Maryland.

"The idea of the study arose because I have a lot of friends who've been on antidepressants and have long-standing interests in hallucinogens. They'd call me up, as their personal pharmacologist, and want to know why they had unusual responses to LSD while taking antidepressants. It turned out that their LSD experience depended on which antidepressant they were taking. Based on these initial reports, I sought to interview people with similar histories by putting ads in the local alternative newspaper, posting notices on Internet newsgroups, and writing an article for a newsletter published by MAPS, the Multidisciplinary Association for Psychedelic Studies. People also contacted me after hearing about the study from friends or health professionals.

"Many people responded, but I could only use reports where there was a *control* condition—either they had taken the same hallucinogen before antidepressant treatment or had friends who had taken the same hallucinogen but were not on antidepressants. Everyone who participated answered a structured questionnaire about their antidepressant treatment, other drugs they regularly used, and past experience with hallucinogens. Then I asked about their experience with a hallucinogen while taking an antidepressant. I was mainly interested in whether they had an increase, a decrease, or no change in their response to the hallucinogen in terms of the time it took to get high, physical effects, hallucinatory effects, psychological effects, the total time they were high, any after-effects or changes in sleep, and their overall impression of the trip.

In a nutshell, people who took Serotonin-selective reuptake inhibitors (SSRIs) or Monoamine oxidase inhibitors (MAOIs) had a decreased response or no response at all to hallucinogens. This is in contrast to what happened when people took tricyclic antidepressants or lithium: these people had a big increase in their response to hallucinogens, often to a very unpleasant degree—this was not a case of having more fun on less acid. Everyone who responded to the survey had been taking antidepressants for at least three to four weeks. This might be important because it takes that much time before certain changes in neurotransmitter systems can occur in the brain after antidepressants are taken. These neurochemical changes also probably account for the three to four week lag time before antidepressants have a therapeutic effect."

Bonson posted her data and the following warning notice on the Internet:

SSRIS

@ **FLUOXETINE (PROZAC®).** Even at doses of this antidepressant ranging from 2-40 mg a day, there was an overall decrease in most effects from LSD (no matter how much acid people took) and a decrease in response to ketamine. There was no change in response to psilocybin, but there does seem to be a decrease in response to MDMA.

@ **SERTRALINE (ZOLOFT®).** The effect with this antidepressant seems dose-dependent. At 50 mg a day, there was no effect on the response to LSD or psilocybin. At 100 mg a day, a decrease in response to LSD and MDMA.

@ **PAROXETINE (PAXIL®).** Decrease in response to LSD.

@ **TRAZODONE (DESYREL®).** Decrease in response to LSD.

TRICYCLICS

@ **IMIPRAMINE (TOFRANIL®).** Increase in response to LSD.

@ **DESIPRAMINE (NORPRAMINE®).** Increase in response to LSD.

@ **CLOMIPRAMINE (ANAFRANIL®).** Increase in response to LSD.

K. BONSON'S ANNOUNCEMENT ON THE INTERNET:

!!!!! NOTE THE RESPONSE TO MDMA !!!!!

Combining an MAO inhibitor plus MDMA has led to hypertensive crisis and a near-fatal response in many people!!! This could be anticipated because MDMA is a [modified] amphetamine, and **stimulants should not be combined with an MAO inhibitor!!!** DO NOT TRY THIS AT HOME!!!

Ⓢ **LITHIUM** (alone or in combination with a tricyclic antidepressant). Increase in response to LSD or psilocybin.

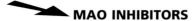**MAO INHIBITORS**

Ⓢ **PHENELZINE (NARDIL®).** Decrease in response to LSD.

"How do we explain these data?" asks Bonson. "This is a bit of a theoretical problem. One would want to say the hallucinogenic response occurs because of $5-HT_2$ stimulation, so there was down-regulation of $5-HT_2$ sites after SSRI antidepressants and MAO inhibitors and this led to elimination of the hallucinogenic response. The problem is, these antidepressants don't always affect the brain this way. A bigger problem is that tricyclic antidepressants are thought to act a lot like SSRIs in their ability to down-regulate $5-HT_2$ sites, so we can't explain why tricyclics seem to increase the response to LSD. We're trying to formulate a theory based on the difference between classes of drugs in terms of their effects on $5-HT_{1A}$ sites and the way different antidepressants affect serotonin levels. Because LSD works at $5-HT_2$ and $5-HT_{1A}$ sites and other receptors, this may explain differences in hallucinogenic responses.

"I am not aware of any reports of adverse reactions between the interaction of antidepressants and hallucinogens, with the exception of MDMA, MAOI and stimulants of any kind," Bonson says. "But that does not preclude the possibility that adverse physical effects could occur. *Psychological* adverse effects definitely happened when people were taking tricyclic antidepressants or lithium and combining it with LSD. They got way higher than they ever expected to. Some people went into fugue states, which means they'd just like take off and end up in another [mental] state. Really bad things happened, like some people couldn't form words and were psychologically just not... at... all... in a place they wanted to be. They effectively had an experience worth two or three times the dose they took. But combining any drug with any other drug opens up unknown risks—we can't predict what will happen."*

---

*If you'd like to contribute a personal anecdote about antidepressants and hallucinogens (other than LSD), write or e-mail: Katherine Bonson, Ph.D., National Institute of Mental Health (NIMH), Building 10, Room 3D41, Bethesda, MD 20892; kbonson@codon.nih.gov

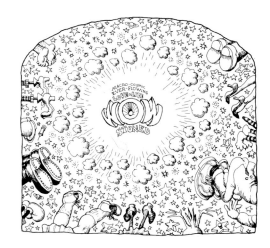

Chapter 9

THE REST OF THE HALLUCINOGENS

MOST HALLUCINOGENS COME from plants. Their use stretches so far back into prehistory that some experts say the very concept of gods comes from ancient tribal shamans who drank psychedelic tea just before reeling into the spirit world. But heck, hallucinogens have been called worse things than the *de facto* source of all religion.

AYAHUASCA

 One of South America's most important lowland hallucinogens is ayahuasca (called *caapi*, *natema*, *pindé* or *yajé*). It's made from the rain forest plants *Banisteriopsis caapi* and *B. inebrians* vine bark and *Psychotria viridis* leaves. The first chemicals isolated from *Banisteriopsis* were compounds called beta-carbolines, which include the hallucinogens harmine, harmaline and tetrahydroharmine.

Ayahuasca's a hallucinogenic tea used in ceremonies in the western Amazon and on the Pacific coasts of Colombia and Ecuador. It causes body and soul to feel like they're separating, and tribes use these sensations to get to what they call the world of the 'little people.'* The tribes call ayahuasca *vine of the soul* and use it to initiate young Indians into manhood, predict the future, settle conflicts, decode enemy plans, cure diseases and mingle with the spirits.

Ayahuasca is made by brewing the stems of *Banisteriopsis* with parts of at least one other plant that contains DMT (often *Psychotria viridis* leaves) to

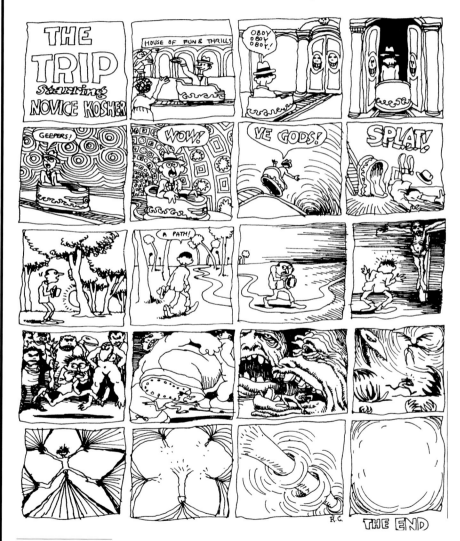

---

*I guess L. Frank Baum (1856–1919) spent some time in the jungle before he went over the rainbow to write about munchkinland in *The Wonderful Wizard of Oz* in 1900 (Mineola, NY: Dover Publications, 1960). Hey look, Frank. They're taking Dorothy!

produce the hallucinogenic tea. DMT isn't active when you take it orally—it usually has to be smoked. But *Banisteriopsis* contains a compound called harmaline that keeps the liver from breaking DMT down and lets it enter the bloodstream when you drink the tea. Harmaline also extends DMT's visionary effects for up to 6 hours.[117] *Banisteriopsis* is supposed to guide the spirits of additive plants and control their effects. Different plants are used for soul travel, telepathy, healing, communicating with spirits, visions, divining the future or learning spirit songs. Some of these are *Psychotria*, *Justicia* and *Tetrapteris;* all contain DMT.[118]

According to ethnopharmacologist Laurent Rivier of the Institut universitaire de médecine légale in Lausanne, Switzerland, "Ayahuasca has a very specific effect on people who take it. They see the scenery around them through a[n optic] blue veil. To people who take mescaline, everything looks like an Aztec design."

◥ CHARLES GROB ON AYAHUASCA

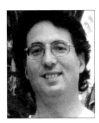

From a July 1996 telephone interview with Dr. Charles Grob, associate professor of psychiatry and pediatrics at the University of California-Los Angeles School of Medicine, and director of the Division of Child and Adolescent Psychiatry at the Harbor-UCLA Medical Center.

"In June 1993 I traveled to Manaus in the Brazilian Amazon to participate in a multidisciplinary, international biomedical-psychiatric investigation of ayahuasca's short- and long-term effects. My main collaborators were Dennis McKenna of the United States, Jace Callaway of Finland and Glacus de Souza Brito of Brazil. We went to study members of the Uniao do Vegetal (UDV), a Brazilian religious movement that got government permission in the late 1980s to use ayahuasca as a ritual sacrament.

"We used a variety of assessment measures on our UDV ayahuasca-using subjects and with a similar number of matched controls who had never used ayahuasca. We did baseline medical evaluations and conducted structured psychiatric diagnostic interviews, personality testing and neuropsychological assessments of memory and concentration. We found interesting contrasts between the two groups, including distinct differences in personality profiles and neuropsychological tests. All our subjects had been UDV members for at least 10 years and ritually drank ayahuasca several times a month over that time, and we wanted to see if there was evidence of negative effects on brain function.

"Not only did we find no such evidence, but on one subtest of the neuropsychological measure, ayahuasca-using subjects scored much better on memory assessment than subjects who didn't use ayahuasca. Another interesting finding was that many of our ayahuasca-using subjects reported alcoholism, drug abuse, violence and antisocial behavior before they joined the UDV. But our psychiatric interviews showed that virtually all this psychopathology stopped after they started participating in the religious ceremonies where ayahuasca is a ritual sacrament.

"We published these findings in the February 1996 issue of the *Journal of Nervous and Mental Disease*. Investigations of ayahuasca's effects on serotonin biochemistry were published December 1994 in *Psychopharmacology*, and of ayahuasca pharmacokinetics [its metabolism and action in the body] in the November 1996 *Journal of Analytical Toxicology*.

"In trying to understand why these subjects—who'd regularly used ayahuasca for 10 or more years—were so high-functioning and without evidence of active pathology, we examined the context in which they take this potent psychedelic. The UDV only use ayahuasca in formal religious ceremonies, never as a recreational drug. The ceremonies are an excellent example of how important it is to account for set and setting in an experiment [especially one that involves psychedelics] to get the best results.

"Another critical factor is that in Brazilian society it's legal [for anyone in Brazil, not just Brazilian citizens] to use ayahuasca for religious purposes. This insures safety and protection under the law, and it's a remarkable historical precedent. The Brazilian government's decision to legally sanction ayahuasca churches is the first time in 1,600 years that a government has legally protected the religious use of psychedelics by its non-indigenous people. That sanction is also essential to conducting a research investigation like ours."

MORNING GLORY SEEDS (*OLOLIUQUI*)[119]

As with the sacred mushrooms, hallucinogenic morning glories are important in the lives of pre-Hispanic Mexicans, but didn't go public until the 20th century. In 1939, botanists collected parts of the *Turbina corymbosa* (morning glory) among the Chinantec and Zapotec people of Oaxaca and cultivated it for hallucinogenic use. The Chinantec name, *T. corymbosa*, means "medicine for divination." It's a vine with lots of long white flowers with round, brown seeds. Users grind 13 seeds and drink them with water or in an alcohol beverage. Morning glory intoxication starts fast, makes some users temporarily giddy and leads to visual hallucinations. Users may be dimly aware of their surroundings and susceptible to suggestion. Visions can be grotesque and usually feature people or events.

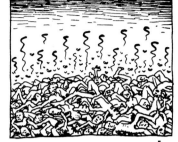

Natives say the intoxication lasts three hours and rarely causes bad after-effects. Healers give *ololiuqui* at night to one person alone in a quiet space. The Aztecs use another morning glory, *Ipomoea violacea*, as a sacred hallucinogen. Its seeds are long, angular and black, and more potent than *T. corymbosa* seeds. Its flowers vary from white to blue or violet and are popular garden plants. The hallucinogenic dose is seven seeds, a multiple of seven or the usual 13. Healers use morning glory to find causes of illness and sometimes lost objects.

Lysergic acid amide [ergine] and lysergic acid hydroethylamide are *ololiuqui's* hallucinogenic elements. Indole alkaloids are isolated from ergot, and *ololiuqui's* molecular structure looks something like the psychoactive elements in psilocybin and the neurotransmitter serotonin. Two to 5 mg of *ololiuqui* is the lowest hallucinogenic dose. That means it's 100 times less potent than LSD, which gives up *its* hallucinogenic effects at 0.05 mg.

◣ PEYOTE (*LOPHOPHORA WILLIAMSii*)[120]

Products of the peyote cactus are major sacraments for the Indians of Mexico. Over the last 100 years, the practice has migrated to North American tribes. The Chichimeca and Toltec tribes probably used peyote 1,900 years before

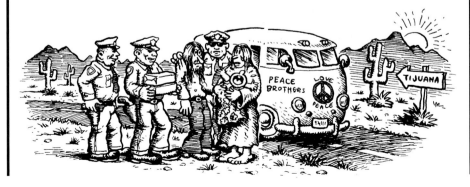

the Europeans landed. That means peyote's economic history extends over two millennia. But archaeological finds in Texas caves and rock shelters include peyote specimens that Indians probably used ceremonially 3,000 years ago. Peyote grows all over Mexico, so scattered tribes probably discovered its psychoactive properties independently. Tribe members cut the peyote cactus's gray-green spineless crowns from the roots and dry them. They store and use the mescal buttons all year.

PEYOTE & THE NATIVE AMERICAN CHURCH
To protect their religious rights, American Indians organized the peyote cult into a legally recognized religious group, the Native American Church. This movement, unknown in the U.S. before 1885, had 13,000 members in 1922. Today, membership is 250,000. U.S. Indians who live far from peyote's natural habitat use mescal buttons, which they legally buy and distribute through the U.S. postal service.

L. WILLIAMSii **WAS THE FIRST** hallucinogenic plant to be chemically analyzed. At the turn of the century, chemists identified its psychoactive element as a crystallized alkaloid. They called the hallucinogen mescaline because they took the alkaloid from a mescal button. Chemists later isolated several alkaloids from peyote and related cacti. Once they found mescaline's chemical structure, chemists could make it in the lab. If you're a chemist it's pretty easy—3,4,5-trimethoxyphenylethylamine. Structurally, mescaline looks like the neurotransmitter norepinephrine.

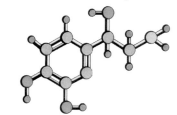

NOREPINEPHRINE (NE)

NATIVE AMERICANS ALSO USE peyote as a medicine, sometimes their only medicine. Primitive societies often believe that supernatural interference causes death or illness. Peyote visions are supposed to put healers face to face with the aforementioned spirits-gone-bad.

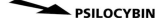 **PSILOCYBIN**

Reverence doesn't quite capture how the pre-Hispanic Mexican Indians feel about sacred mushrooms. The Aztecs called the mushrooms *Teonanacatl* (divine flesh) and used them only in the holiest ceremonies. Until the 1930s, few people outside Mexico knew about hallucinogenic

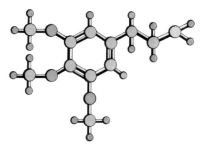

MESCALINE

mushrooms, their chemistry or their role in Mexican culture. In the late 1930s, researchers collected two sacred mushroom species and associated them with a modern Mexican mushroom ceremony. Later fieldwork turned up 25 or so species; 12 belonged to the genus *Psilocybe* and produced the most important mushrooms. Mexican natives have held mushroom ceremonies for centuries. Archaeological evidence from Guatemala dates them from the first millennium B.C.[121]

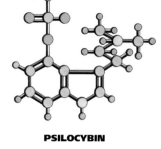

PSILOCYBIN

TEONANACATL are hallucinogenic thanks to the alkaloids psilocybin and psilocin. Psilocybin, a chemical component of psilocin that usually shows up only in trace elements, is the main psychoactive element in *teonanacatl*. Psilocybin and psilocin are indole alkaloids and have a close chemical link to the neurotransmitter serotonin, which may be involved in the biochemistry of things like sleep, appetite and mood.

In the mid-1950s, Albert Hofmann isolated, concentrated and purified the mushrooms' psychoactive element into the colorless crystal compounds psilocybin and psilocin. He and his team published the results in

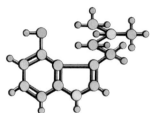

PSILOCIN

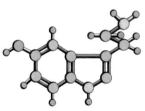

SEROTONIN (5-HT)

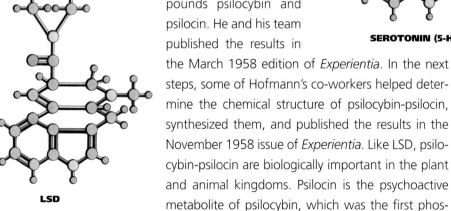

LSD

the March 1958 edition of *Experientia*. In the next steps, some of Hofmann's co-workers helped determine the chemical structure of psilocybin-psilocin, synthesized them, and published the results in the November 1958 issue of *Experientia*. Like LSD, psilocybin-psilocin are biologically important in the plant and animal kingdoms. Psilocin is the psychoactive metabolite of psilocybin, which was the first phosphoric-acid-containing indole compound discovered in nature. Psilocin decomposes when it's exposed to air; psilocybin is stable. Features common to psilocybin-psilocin and LSD are their chemical structures and psychoactive effects.

Psilocybin-psilocin also look a lot like serotonin and, like LSD, they block the effects of serotonin in pharmacological experiments. Psilocybin is hallucinogenic at 6-12 mg. The average psychoactive dose of psilocybin or psilocin in humans is 10 mg. That means LSD is more than 100 times stronger, and its effects last 9-12 hours compared with 4-6 hours for psilocybin-psilocin.[122]

DMT[123]

Chemically, DMT is N,N-dimethyl-3-(2-aminoethyl) indole, a white, pungent-smelling, crystalline solid that dissolves in organic solvents and aqueous acids but not in water. It's a hallucinogenic component of several snuffs used by South American natives. The parent compound tryptamine *and* the enzyme that converts it to DMT exist in humans. So far, no one knows the origins or functions of endogenous DMT. There's lots of evidence that DMT forms in the body, and trace amounts have been found in the blood and urine of healthy people and schizophrenics.

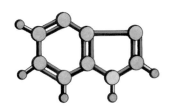

INDOLE RING

In users, an increase in excreted 5-hydroxyindoleacetic acid (5-HIAA), a major serotonin metabolite, suggests serotonin is involved in DMT action. DMT doesn't work if it's taken orally unless it's combined with a monoamine oxidase (MAO) inhibitor like harmaline, an ingredient with DMT in ayahuasca; and iproniazid, the first drug to be used as an antidepressant (1956). If DMT's injected into a muscle, there's an abrupt level of activity at 30 mg and a complete psychedelic experience at 50 to 70 mg. The high comes on fast. Within 5 minutes pupils dilate, heartbeat speeds up, blood pressure rises. In 10-15 minutes you've got visual distortions whether your eyes are open or closed, and lots of movement in the visual field.

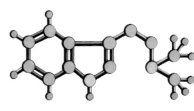

DMT

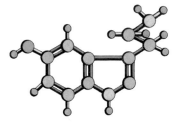

SEROTONIN (5-HT)

You have trouble expressing thoughts. You have the attention span of a golden retriever. You're euphoric and screaming with laughter. *Or...* something goes terribly wrong and your paranoid ideation turns anxiety and feelings of doom into full-blown panic. But, one way or another, it's mostly gone in an hour.

DMT's active at 30 mg when it's inhaled (snuffed, snorted), but it comes on in 10 seconds, you're high for two to three minutes, and you touch down 10 minutes after ignition and launch. Intramuscuarly, 1.0 mg/kg or so of

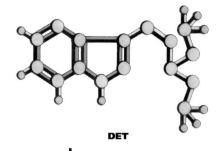

DET

DMT is hallucinogenic. There's no cross-tolerance[*] with LSD, and repeated use doesn't lead to physical or psychological addiction. DMT is a powerful hallucinogen chemically related to psilocybin and more distantly to LSD. Side effects include stimulation and tactile hallucinations while tripping. At least two synthetic drugs that are structurally similar to DMT are psychedelic. N,N-diethyltryptamine

(DET[**]) is active at the same dose as DMT and the effects last a little longer—1.5 to 2 hours. At 15 to 30 mg, the lowest effective dose, N,N-dipropyltryptamine (DPT) lasts 1.5 to 2 hours; at 60 to 150 mg, it lasts 4 to 6 hours. DET and DPT are milder than DMT and, like DMT, have to be smoked or injected.

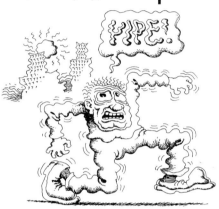

OTHER HALLUCINOGENS

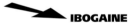 **IBOGAINE**

Ibogaine is a psychoactive indole alkaloid from root bark of the rain forest

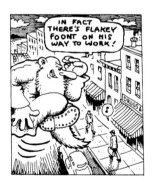

shrub *Tabernanthe iboga.* Like other hallucinogens, it can be made synthetically. Natives of Western Africa cultivate and use iboga as a stimulant, aphrodisiac, hunting aid and, in higher doses, as a sacrament in religious rituals. Iboga is hallucinogenic and such a powerful central nervous system stimulant that users can exert themselves physically for a long time. The body feels light or like it's floating, and users see color spec-

---

[*]Cross-tolerance between drugs means that people who develop tolerance (need higher and higher doses to get to the same level) to one drug will also be tolerant to the other, even if they've never taken the second drug. It happens a lot with benzodiazepines like Valium and barbiturates like Seconal. From Snyder, 164.

[**]In the United States in the late 1950s, Stephen Szára, who synthesized DMT and reported its psychoactive properties in 1956, developed diethyltryptamine (DET), a psychoactive derivative of DMT.

tra (rainbow effects) in surrounding objects. Iboga has such a strong impact on motor activity that in tribal initiation ceremonies, the initiates eventually collapse and have to be carried to a special house or forest shelter. While an initiate is cognitively unavailable, the tribe believes his "shadow" (soul) leaves his body to wander with ancestors in the land of the dead. Tribe mem-

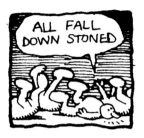

bers think of iboga as a "generic ancestor." Sorcerers in the Bwiti cult and other secret societies in Gabon use it to query the spirit world, and cult leaders use it to get advice from ancestors. Seeing spectra tells them they're approaching the realms of ancestors and gods. Time stretches out and the spiritual trip may seem to take days. Large

doses can crosswire senses like hearing, smell and taste. Moods can run from fear to euphoria.[124]

Researchers identified ibogaine as the bark's main psychoactive agent in 1901, then studied its central nervous system effects and cardiovascular pharmacology through the early 20th century. In the 1950s, CIBA Geigy Pharmaceutical Co. investigated ibogaine's ability to lower blood pressure. At the same time, some French mountaineers used ibogaine on long expeditions to fight hunger and fatigue. And, like practically every other known chemical compound on earth, ibogaine eventually showed up in the late '60s drug culture.[125]

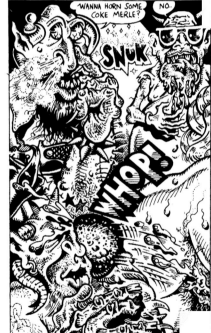

In 1962-3 Howard Lotsof, now head of a company called NDA International, held a series of group experiments to show ibogaine's effect on cocaine and heroin addiction. In 1969 and 1973, psychiatrist Claudio Naranjo was first to report using ibogaine as a hallucinogen in experimental psychotherapy. Then in 1985 Lotsof applied for utility patents on ibogaine. The U.S. Patent and Trade Office grants utility patents to anyone who invents or discovers a new and useful process, or a new and useful process improvement.[126]

Lotsof received U.S. patent 4,499,096 on ibogaine as a treatment for opiate-narcotic addiction (1985); U.S. patent 4,587,243 on ibogaine as a treatment for cocaine addiction (1986); and U.S. patent 5,152,994 on ibogaine as a treatment for polydrug dependence disorders (1992).

Lotsof says he uses ibogaine to interrupt chemical dependence—usually an initial treatment, then occasional re-treatment for up to two years. Supposedly, patients stay clean for 3-6 months after one dose; 10 percent stay clean for 2 or more years from one treatment; and 10 percent use drugs again 2 weeks after treatment. He says people who use ibogaine this way usually have 4-6 hours of something like dreams about past events, a period of thinking about the events, a period of stimulation, and sleep, then they wake up with no desire to use the drug they were using. But responses to ibogaine are different for everyone.[127]

MARK MOLLIVER ON IBOGAINE

From a February 1996 personal interview with Mark Molliver, a professor in the Department of Neuroscience and Neurology at Johns Hopkins University, Baltimore, Maryland. He's spent 20 years studying mechanisms of drug-induced neuronal injury and how mood-changing drugs work in the brain.

"Ibogaine is a very powerful hallucinogen that's being evaluated for [use with cocaine abusers]. The story behind it is that a student, Howard Lotsof in New York, was in a drug-using group 10 or 12 years ago. I guess they got tired of the usual drugs and wanted something more exciting. They heard about a drug used by pygmy natives in Central Africa, the Congo. It's described as a hallucinogenic tea, but it's a ritual drug used in religious ceremonies. Tribe members also use the drug to initiate young males as tribal warriors and hunters. Lotsof got some of the tea and drank it. He said he woke up the next morning and had lost his interest in drugs. He gave it to several friends who said they had the same experience. Lotsof thought it had a potent antiaddictive effect [which hasn't yet been scientifically established]. He patented ibogaine to treat addiction to other drugs, formed a company to represent and market it, and lobbied effectively to pressure government [agencies] to develop it as an addiction treatment. He's a committed individual and believes it works. I'm not sure. It certainly has potent effects.

"We've been studying ibogaine for several years and find that it also has some toxicity. It can cause brain damage in certain regions [of rat and monkey brains] and we're very interested in it from that point of view. Experimentally we've looked at it at somewhat higher doses than are used [by people]. In rats ibogaine causes degeneration of certain nerve cells in the cerebellum. We've also given it to monkeys and found that at higher doses it has similar effects. NIDA was developing it for addiction treatment and they asked us to look at it. We reported this [toxic effect] to NIDA and FDA, and NIDA decided to back off. FDA is still interested and authorized [researchers at the] University of Miami to run a small clinical trial at very low doses.

"We're still very interested in further studies to find out where ibogaine acts in the brain. We have some ideas—we know where it acts in some places but not everywhere. I and a colleague, Elizabeth O'Hearn, both have grants to study the effects of ibogaine and its mechanisms of action. We're planning to study it for several years in the future, partly because it's interesting in terms of its relevance to understanding addiction, and because it causes brain damage [in rat and monkey brains]. It's given us a model system for studying a type of drug-induced brain damage we call *excitotoxicity*. Ibogaine's an excitatory compound and an extremely potent hallucinogen—one of the most potent in terms of the nature and types of hallucinations it produces. The Bwiti tribe in Africa has a whole folklore about the hallucinations—it's part of their religion. They believe when you take it, you go back into the past and see your ancestors and the whole development of the culture. Your whole perspective of life allegedly changes.

"Ibogaine is closely related to another hallucinogen, harmaline, from South American rain forests at about the same latitude. Harmaline is related to DMT and it's usually taken in a [tea] mixture with DMT called ayahuasca. Someone recently uncovered a story that ibogaine and particularly harmaline were used in ancient Persia—they discovered ancient documents describing its use at the beginnings of history. We heard from another group of people that they were taking people to Brazil to take harmaline as a spiritual and antiaddictive experience. That was independent confirmation, based on this ritual story, that ibogaine and harmaline are powerful hallucinogens. Both have antiaddictive effects and both cause the same toxicity.

"With both drugs we found that in the cerebellum there are large principle neurons called Purkinje cells, named after Jan Purkinje who first described these cells. After taking a large dose of either drug, rows of Purkinje cells degenerated. [Like dominoes], rows of cells, columns of cells, from front to back, are completely wiped out. Purkinje cells are the principle neurons in the cerebellum. The cerebellum is involved in coordinating movement, but I think right now it's beginning to emerge that the cerebellum's also involved in learning and a number of cognitive functions. It's just beginning to be understood.

"The cerebellum is like a large sheet, what we call grey matter, where neurons are arranged in little modular circles. It receives input from all over the brain and from all sensory modalities, integrates them and generates an output. And it's the Purkinje cells that integrate signals in the cerebellum and generate an output that goes to other parts of the brain, particularly to the cerebral cortex. So we think some caution should be used in taking these drugs. What we have found is that in monkeys ibogaine is less toxic—[but] you still get some toxicity and it's still potentially dangerous. And that was largely why NIDA decided to back off from promoting ibogaine [but not from studying it]. NIDA's Basic Science Division still supports our studies but the Medications Development Division decided not to invest more funds."

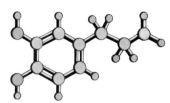

DOPAMINE

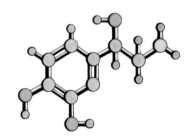

NOREPINEPHRINE

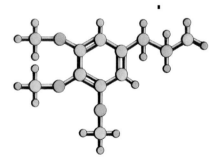

MESCALINE

 MESCALINE[128]

Mescaline (3,4,5-trimethoxyphenethylamine) is a white substance whose crystals are long, needle-shaped structures. Dopamine and norepinephrine have the same carbon skeleton. Mescaline's molecular weight is 211.25—that's 62.54 percent carbon, 8.11 percent hydrogen, 6.63 percent nitrogen and 22.72 percent oxygen, also written $C_{11}H_{17}NO_3$. Its main metabolite is 3,4,5-trimethoxyphenylacetic acid. Mescaline can be modified to become lots of similar compounds but it's only psychoactive if you add a methyl group (NH_3) at the alpha-carbon site (just like you thought). Mescaline-related hallucinogens are DMA, TMA-2, para-DOT, DOM (also called STP and developed in the 1960s by Alexander Shulgin), DOB and 2C-B.

ALEXANDER SHULGIN ON MESCALINE

from *PIHKAL (Phenethylamines I Have Known and Loved): A Chemical Love Story* (Berkeley: Trasform Press; 1991), html version. http://www.hyperreal.ncom/drugs/pihkal/index.html. Used with permission.

DOSE: 200-400 mg as a sulfate salt, 178-256 mg as a hydrochloride salt.

DURATION: 10-12 hours.

QUALITATIVE COMMENTS

300 MG: I would have liked to, and was expecting to, have an exciting visual day, but I seemed to be unable to escape self-analysis. At the peak of the experience, I was quite intoxicated and hyper with energy, so that it was not hard to move around. I was quite restless. But I spent most of the day in considerable agony, trying to break through without success. I learned a great deal about myself and my inner workings.

350 MG: Once I got through the nausea stage, I ventured outdoors and was aware of an intensification of color and a considerable change in the texture of the cloth of my shirt and in the concrete of the sidewalk, and in the flowers and leaves that were handed me by an observer. I experienced the desire to laugh hysterically at what I could only describe as the completely ridiculous state of the entire world.

400 MG: During the initial phase of the intoxication (2-3 hours), everything seemed to have a humorous interpretation. People's faces are in caricature, small cars seem to be chasing big cars, and all cars coming toward me seem to have faces... A remarkable effect of this drug is the extreme empathy felt for all small things; a stone, a flower, an insect. I 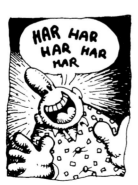 believe it would be impossible to harm anything—to commit an overt harmful or painful act on anyone or anything is beyond one's capabilities... I found color perception to be the most striking aspect of the experience. The slightest difference of shade could be amplified to extreme contrast. Many subtle hues became phosphorescent in intensity. Saturated colors were often unchanged but surrounded by cascades of new colors tumbling over the edges.

DOM

According to Alexander and Ann Shulgin, "Mescaline is one of the oldest known psychedelics. It's the major active component of the small dumpling cactus, peyote. It grows wild in the southwestern United States and northern Mexico, where native Indians have used it for centuries as a sacrament in religious ceremonies. The cactus, *Lophophora williamsii* or *Anhalonium lewinii*, is immediately recognizable by its small round shape and tufts of soft fuzz instead of conventional spines. During ceremonies, tribe members take 2-24 hard tops, called buttons.[129]

"Mescaline has always been the standard against which all other compounds are viewed. Even the U.S. Chemical Warfare group, in human studies of several substituted phenethylamines, used mescaline as the reference material for quantitative and qualitative comparisons. The Edgewood Arsenal code number for mescaline was EA-1306. All psychedelics are characterized by properties that are something like 'twice the potency of mescaline' or 'twice as long-lived as mescaline.'[130]

"This simple drug is the central prototype against which everything else is measured. The earliest studies with the 'psychotomimetic amphetamines' had quantitative psychological numbers attached that read as mescaline units. Mescaline was cast in concrete as being active at the 3.75 mg/kg level. That means 300 mg for a 170-pound person. If a new compound proved

MESCALINE

active at 30 mg, an MU level of 10 went into the published literature. The behavioral biologists were happy because now they had numbers to represent psychological properties. But, in truth, none of this represented the magic of this material, the nature of the experience itself."[131]

KETAMINE[132]

In 1963, the search for a safe general anesthetic led pharmacologists to phencyclidines like PCP (angel dust). They were okay as anesthetics but tended to cause trance-like psychotic reactions in patients. More research produced ketamine, introduced in 1965 by pharmacologists at the University of Michigan. Ketamine wasn't perfect but it produced less obvious psychotic reactions.

Parke-Davis mass-produced it as Ketalar, a safe general anesthetic with a fast onset and recovery and a wide safety margin. Ketamine was used heavily in Vietnam. Chemically, it's 2-(2-chlorophenyl)-2-(methylamino)-cyclohexa-none—a dissociative anesthetic used in animals and humans. Psychologically it's very safe. Physically, people who take 100 mg lose coordination. The dis-

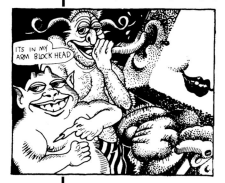

sociative part means the mind seems separate from the body. In people, this sometimes causes hallucinations and the feeling of entering another reality; a benzodiazapine like Versed is used with it.

Ketamine's most important characteristic is that it causes only mild respiratory depression and usually doesn't affect cough and gag reflexes. Unlike other strong anesthetic drugs, patients who take it won't aspirate their own saliva. Ketamine is available nonmedically as ketamine hydrochloride. Some major chemical houses sell it for $10 a gram in doses that range from 100-500 mg. It's usually given intravenously or intramuscularly. Street users snort it or drink it in a solution. Ketamine HCl is available in 100-mg-per-ml injectable doses under the trade name Vetalar from Parke-Davis and Ketaset from Bristol.

At the beginning of 1996, the only scientific researcher who was directly investigating the therapeutic potential of a psychedelic was Dr. Evgeny Krupitsky, chief researcher at the Leningrad Regional Dispensary of Narcology. Krupitsky had been researching ketamine for 10 years to treat alcoholism and wanted to expand his research to treating post-traumatic stress disorder (PTSD) and drug addiction. In 1996, he got a grant from the National Institute on Alcoholism and Alcohol Abuse

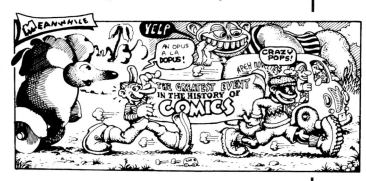

(NIAAA) to fund a ketamine study to be conducted with John Krystal at Yale Medical School. The study would determine ketamine's mechanism of action at the neurotransmitter level. Ketamine is chemically related to PCP, an unpredictable street drug whose effects include bad trips, psychotic reactions and extreme violence in users. Ketamine is safer than PCP, which is no longer used medically. Street users heat liquid ketamine to form a white powder, then smoke or snort it. The effects last about an hour. Ketamine is nontoxic and has been used in experimental psychotherapy.

PCP[133]

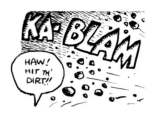

Phencyclidine (PCP, angel dust) was synthesized in 1958. In 1960 and 1963, Parke, Davis & Co. got patent rights to use PCP medically as an anesthetic. Pharmacologically, PCP is a pseudo-hallucinogen with downer characteristics that has bizarre effects on some users. Its synthesis was published in 1965, but there was no real pharmacological basis for producing designer PCP until the original patent and later studies were available. PCP first appeared on the streets in 1967, then dropped out of sight.

The DEA, then the Bureau of Narcotics and Dangerous Drugs, listed PCP as a drug of abuse in the late '60s. In the early 1970s, phencyclidine reappeared on the streets, this time as a drug of deceit. Since it's easily and cheaply synthesized in clandestine labs, it's often sold on the street as THC, cannabinol, mescaline, psilocybin, LSD, amphetamine, cocaine, Hawaiian woodrose and other psychedelics. In one study only 3 percent of analyzed street drug samples that contained PCP actually sold as PCP. THC, which isn't usually available on the street, is the most common misrepresentation.

MDA[134]

Chemically, MDA is 3,4-methylenedioxyamphetamine, the parent chemical of MDMA (N-methyl-3,4-methylenedioxyamphetamine). No wonder recreational drug users give them names like *ecstasy*. It's active dose is 80-160 mg and it lasts 8-12 hours. On the street, people who buy MDMA often get MDE or MDA instead. MDA has a long history of use and abuse. It was one of the CIA and Army potential truth drugs of abuse, tested randomly on anyone who'd stand still long enough.

One 1953 case involved MDA and a psychiatric patient named Howard Blauer. Back then, the Army contracted with several physicians at the New York State Psychiatric Institute to study all the fascinating new chemicals from Edgewood Arsenal. Among them was EA-1298-MDA. They used it intravenously on Blauer a few times, then one day he got that really big injection. MDA/EA-1298 is psychoactive at 80-160 mg, but they gave him 500 mg—truly a killer dose—and that's the last time Howard Blauer tested anything for anyone.[135]

MDA's been used in medical environments as a diet pill and an experimental treatment for depression. Several medical reports and a book, *The Healing Journey* by psychiatrist Claudio Naranjo[136], describe MDA's psychotherapeutic value. In the late 1960s, MDA was popular on the streets; users called it the hug drug. In the late 1960s, it was easy to get huge quantities because MDA was still available as a research chemical from scientific supply houses, sold cheaply—$9.50 for 10 g in 1966-67, so about 9.5 cents* a dose[137] as 3,4-methylenedioxyamphetamine.[138]

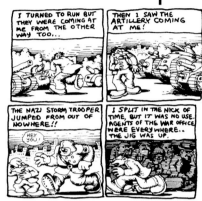

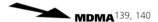 **MDMA**[139, 140]

In 1913 the German company Merck patented MDMA, but never marketed the drug. MDMA resurfaced in 1953 as part of (what else?) an Army interrogation-drug testing program. Meanwhile, in northern California, Alexander Shulgin earned a doctorate in biochemistry at the University of California at

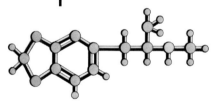

MDMA

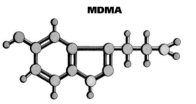

SEROTONIN

Berkeley and went to work for Dow Chemical as a research chemist. After he invented a profitable insecticide, Dow gave him a free hand and his own lab. Shulgin decided to study psychedelic drugs. Later, when Dow realized it held patents to a popular street drug, Shulgin's association with Dow ended. Afterward he tested new compounds on himself and friends for years, then got federal approval to work with hallucinogens and other Schedule I drugs. He specialized in phenethylamines like mescaline and MDMA, and recorded the effects of every compound in the phenethylamine family. He's been called the stepfather of MDMA.[141] His book, *PIHKAL—Phenethylamines I Have Known And Loved*, details the workings and

---

*Huh. When was the 'cents' symbol exiled from the keyboard?

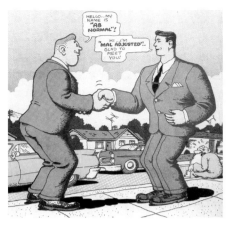

effects of 179 psychoactive drugs, including MDMA.

In the brain, MDMA causes a big release of 5-HT from presynaptic vesicles, increasing brain levels of serotonin. But researchers don't know much yet about long-term psychological and physical consequences of depletion on people. For more than 30 years Shulgin clinically studied psychedelic phenethylamine derivatives and created the largest single database on their human psychopharmacology. MDMA also came closest to his goal of finding a new therapeutic drug.[142] Psychotherapists who used MDMA in treatment liked it because it reduced anxiety and gave patients a calmer understanding of their problems.

In 1984, MDMA was still legal in the United States. American students called it ecstasy and tossed it down like Jolt Cola. This and the growing blatant use of ecstasy prompted DEA to outlaw MDMA. In 1985 a small group of MDMA fans sued DEA to keep the drug legal. The controversy went coast to coast faster than a retrovirus, creating an even bigger demand for MDMA. But several years before ecstasy hit the media, a group of clandestine U.S. drug manufacturers made a flawed batch of China White—synthetic heroin sold to junkies as a legal substitute. The batch had a chemical impurity that in some users caused a form of brain damage like Parkinson's disease. So Congress passed a law that let DEA

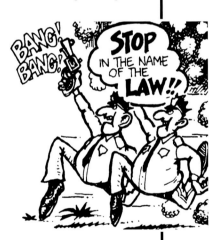

put an emergency ban on any drug it thought might harm the public. In July 1985, DEA used the law to ban MDMA, which abruptly rose to Schedule I on the DEA's list of controlled substances.

Like most kinds of prohibition, the MDMA ban cut clinical research off at the knees while MDMA stayed freely available on the streets. The ban lasted a year. Meanwhile, a hearing was set up to decide what permanent measures should be taken against the drug. The judge recommended scheduling MDMA as a drug that could be manufactured and used in research and by

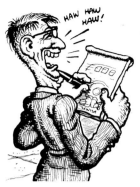

prescription. Instead, DEA kept MDMA in Schedule I and supporters challenged the move in the Federal Court of Appeals. Their objection was overturned in March 1988.

Back on the West Coast, in October 1994, DEA and other federal, state and local agents showed up unannounced, with search warrants, at Shulgin's home in Lafayette, California. Thirty agents and eight vehicles (including a fire engine and a squadron of marked police cars) dropped in to conduct a routine (for them) administrative inspection. They wanted to make sure Shulgin was complying with the rules that governed his DEA license to possess and work with Schedule I substances. When the agents found what they determined to be administrative and environmental infractions, DEA fined him $25,000. As part of the final arrangements, Shulgin gave his license back to them. From their retirement fund, the Shulgins paid $40,000 in fines and legal fees.[143]

Four researchers on
ECSTASY AND BRAIN CELL DESTRUCTION

MARK MOLLIVER ON MDA & MDMA

From a February 1996 personal interview with Mark Molliver, Ph.D., professor, Department of Neuroscience and Neurology, Johns Hopkins University, Baltimore.

"LSD-like hallucinogens are probably not addictive but amphetamines are, and they're often classed as hallucinogens. MDA and MDMA are very mild hallucinogens. An associated group called DOB and DOI are amphetamine-related like MDA and are quite potent hallucinogens. Amphetamines vary in their effects. If you plug different chemical groups in at different sites on the molecule, you change its properties. Classic amphetamine primarily releases dopamine and some norepinephrine in the brain. That's a potent stimulant but not much in the way of a hallucinogen. Chemists have found that if you put the right chemical substituents on an amphetamine, it becomes very hallucinogenic.

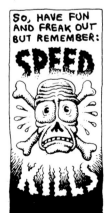

"The hallucinogenic change usually relates to modifying the action of the drug to act more at serotonin sites than at dopamine or norepinephrine. LSD acts at serotonin receptors, and amphetamines modified to act at serotonin receptors are more hallucinogenic. [Biochemist and researcher Alexander] Shulgin has done a lot of the work—he's the ultimate drug designer—putting these groups on different sites then looking at their hallucinogenic effects. Other people have done the receptor studies—to see which receptors are active. That correlates well with hallucinogenic properties at serotonin receptors. So, for example, MDA-ecstasy-related drugs act primarily by releasing serotonin in the brain [this is the 'other' effect of MDA and MDMA that separated them from other hallucinogens and prompted Dave Nichols at Purdue to rename them entactogens].

"At one time I collaborated with Ray Fuller, the person at Eli Lilly who developed Prozac. Prozac also increases the effects of serotonin and is a powerful antidepressant with very few side effects. The [older] antidepressants have all kinds of side effects. Prozac blocks the effects of drugs [like MDA and MDMA] that release serotonin, because they all act at the same site as Prozac—they bind to [serotonin's] reuptake carrier. But MDA and MDMA do more than release serotonin—they cause serotonin nerves to degenerate. Prozac completely blocks that. It prevents the toxicity. We've considered recommending Prozac for treating MDMA overdoses. Prozac actually displaces the other drugs from their sites of action, protecting nerve cells from their effects. If you go in within 12 or 18 hours, you can protect nerve cells against damage from MDA.

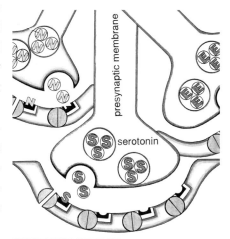

SEROTONIN NEURON

"Another drug—dexfenfluramine—has a similar action to MDA. It's an amphetamine derivative that's being promoted as a diet drug and has the same toxicity as MDMA, causing degeneration of serotonin terminals in the brain. It releases serotonin from all the terminals. Then, if you wait about 24 hours, the nerve terminals that release serotonin go on to degenerate. If you come in with Prozac in the interim, you can displace the drug and protect the nerve terminals.

"[After the neuron fires and serotonin crosses the synaptic gap to bind to the receptor,] an uptake carrier draws serotonin back up into the terminal, mainly to stop the neurotransmission process. So there's a pulse of serotonin, it's removed probably by reuptake (the principal way serotonin, norepinephrine and dopamine are removed from the synapse) and metabolized inside the nerve terminal.

"We don't know exactly how the amphetamines that release serotonin work, but they bind to the uptake part and cause release at the terminal. After binding, they probably get inside and cause the terminal to release all its stored transmitter so it's completely empty. Now Prozac binds to that transporter with very high affinity, knocking everything else off. The amphetamine is displaced and its effect is terminated. Prozac blocks reuptake, so whatever's out there isn't going to be taken back up, but no more is released. It doesn't prevent just any release—natural release might still occur—but excessive release caused by the amphetamine stops. After 24 or 36 hours, [the serotonin terminal] starts to degenerate. Amphetamine works at dopamine and norepinephrine terminals. There's some evidence it causes dopamine terminals to degenerate but it's not so clear-cut, nothing like the effects of MDA and related drugs. Those unequivocally cause massive destruction of all serotonin terminals."

GEORGE RICAURTE ON MDMA

From a March 1996 personal interview with George Ricaurte, Ph.D., Johns Hopkins Bayview campus. He's investigated MDMA for nine years and has studied MDA, amphetamines and many similar drugs.

"The usual dose for MDMA is 1-1.5 tablets, or approximately 75-150 mg, This is the dose a person would take to experience the drug's effects. It's important to draw a distinct line between MDMA's pharmacology, its psychoactive effects, and the neurotoxic effects MDMA is known to produce in laboratory animals. The neurotoxic effects are long-term effects that we believe are related to MDMA-induced damage of serotonin axons and axon terminals.

"If we give animals MDMA and examine serotonin neurons in their brains, we find a number of markers for serotonin neurons are markedly reduced for 2-8 weeks. Beyond 8-12 weeks, there's evidence the damaged serotonin neuron can recover and begin to regrow. But by one year in most rats that have [had] MDMA, one sees what appears to be—although this is not yet entirely clear—a normal serotonin reinnervation pattern [the nerve terminals start to grow back]. If you do the same study in [monkeys], you see that MDMA-treated monkeys show marked deficits in the serotonin axon markers for as long as 18 months beyond drug exposure to MDMA. Normal reinnervation patterns have not been established 18 months after drug exposure. We're in the process of carrying out studies that characterize this abnormal reinnervation pattern in the monkey.

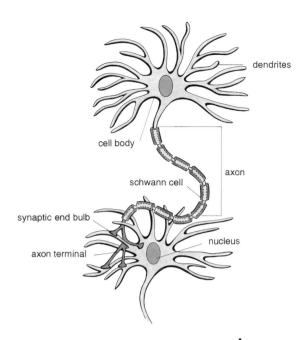

"What seems to happen is that serotonin axons that innervate distant brain areas like the dorsal neocortex don't grow back, whereas axons that innervate closer regions, like the hypothalamus, seem to grow back in excess. So in the long term one sees a marked serotonin deficiency in brain areas like the dorsal neocortex, and a significant excess of serotonin in areas like the hypothalamus, which is closer to the nerve-cell bodies that give rise to these axons. That's a simplified description of the changes seen in MDMA-treated monkeys. These need further study... we need to further identify factors that determine why some serotonin axon projections grow back and others don't.

"A major question in the field is, *What does serotonin do in the central nervous system?* We don't really understand the functional role of serotonin in *any* area of the brain. We have some ideas but... until we gain a more precise understanding of what serotonin does in particular brain regions, it would be premature to speculate about what deficiencies or excesses of serotonin in a particular region of the monkey brain might mean in terms of functional consequences to the animal [and then to humans]. So far, the observations I've described have only been made in experimental animals. Whether these findings generalize to people who use MDMA is under active investigation.

"At present we're conducting a study in people who report a history of extensive MDMA use. We are bringing those people to Johns Hopkins. To participate in the study, people have to agree to remain drug-free, including MDMA, for at least two weeks before coming for the study. While they're in Baltimore, we try to study the status of serotonin neurons in their brains and compare our findings with people who haven't been exposed to MDMA.

"We have seen people who have developed neuropsychiatric problems after using MDMA [but] they comprise a distinct minority. They appear to have developed problems because they were somehow susceptible to MDMA. Most people we enroll in the study appear normal. But it would be premature at this stage to conclude that there are no functional consequences of MDMA in these individuals because it's difficult to ascertain functional consequences of serotonin deficiency. In instances where we have a clue that serotonin is involved in a function, that function is inherently difficult to measure. For example, we think serotonin is involved in mood regulation. How do you measure that in an animal? How do you measure it in people?

"I often hear the argument that if all these people have taken MDMA and seem normal, MDMA must not produce neurotoxic effects. But it is important to recognize that our measures of brain serotonin function are imperfect.

"One thing we hope to learn from MDMA is how it destroys or damages serotonin axons and axon terminals. Perhaps we can get some insight into the mechanisms that underlie degeneration of serotonin neurons in human diseases like Parkinson's disease (which also affects dopamine) and related neurodegenerating conditions. For many years we thought neurons in the CNS couldn't grow back after injury. Now we know that under certain conditions they can; for example, after MDMA injury.

"[People who use MDMA] ought to be careful because they risk damaging serotonin neurons in their brains. How can one be careful? Given the experimental data, if you want to reduce your risk of incurring serotonin neurotoxicity, you would do well to use the lowest amount of MDMA possible, as infrequently as possible—assuming what you buy on the street is pure MDMA. [In terms of unsupervised use of MDMA,] I'd be careful as to how I used MDMA..

"I don't mean to be alarmist. As yet we don't know conclusively that MDMA is neurotoxic in humans. If we did, we wouldn't be doing the studies. But I do know about the effects of MDMA in animals... and my opinion is that in MDMA we have a very interesting psychoactive drug that is a very potent serotonin neurotoxin that could well be harmful to serotonin neurons in human brains. I define MDMA neurotoxicity as the drug's propensity to destroy—prune—serotonin axons and axon terminals. No more, no less."*

CHARLES GROB ON MDMA

> Charles Grob, M.D., associate professor of psychiatry and pediatrics, the University of California-Los Angeles School of Medicine; director, Division of Child and Adolescent Psychiatry, the Harbor-UCLA Medical Center.

"In 1994 our research team at the Harbor-UCLA Medical Center started a Phase 1 investigation on the effects of MDMA in 18 normal volunteers who'd taken the drug before. In our Clinical Research Unit in the hospital, we held three experimental sessions. In two of the sessions the subjects got doses of MDMA, and in one they got an inactive placebo. We used a randomized, double-blind method where neither subjects or staff knew what they were getting or giving in any session. Before they became part of the study, we screened the subjects for medical, psychiatric or substance abuse disorders. Before their first experimental drug session, the subjects had baseline neuropsychological tests, single-photon-emission computed tomography brain scans and magnetic resonance spectroscopy [so researchers could tell if the subjects' pre- and post-experiment readings differed].

"In the experimental sessions we drew blood every 30 minutes for pharmacokinetic assays. At 15-minute intervals we took physiological vital signs including temperature, blood pressure and cardiac rate, and several subjective psychological rating scales [subjects answer questions during the experiment about feelings and perceptions]. The most valuable self-report instrument was the Altered States Graphic Profile [ASGP—see "Other Stuff"], developed by Ralph Metzner, a researcher in this field for 35 years.

"One thing I believe we showed with this study is that it's possible to get permission [from DEA and FDA] to investigate the effects of MDMA in human volunteers, and that it's possible to conduct such a study safely. For some time it seemed impossible to investigate MDMA because of its association with psychedelics and because some researchers think it may be neurotoxic. Lots of people used to think this work was potentially valuable but

---

*Want to participate in the study? Call (410) 550-0993 and speak with research coordinator Linda Klein, who can fax you the study requirements.

impossible because of the political climate. Given that we've been able to get all the approvals and conduct the study safely, we hope other reputable research groups will apply for permission to extend an important, neglected area of investigation.

"We did the Phase 1 MDMA study for two reasons. The first is that there are tremendous public health implications of a substance that hundreds of thousands—even millions—of mostly young people worldwide have taken, that's potentially very risky, and that's never been methodologically studied in human populations. The second is that intriguing anecdotal reports suggest MDMA may have a role in [psychiatric] treatment. A Phase 1 study that establishes safety parameters is needed to develop studies for assessing MDMA's value as a treatment [for mental disorders].

"One interesting thing we observed in our subjects that's relevant to concerns about MDMA risks involves MDMA's effect on body temperature. About 20 deaths have been reported to date, mostly in Great Britain, caused by malignant hyperthermic response [lethally high body temperatures] in people who took MDMA. Most cases occurred during raves [marathon dances] and seemed associated with dehydration in people who danced all night in badly ventilated clubs. Some temperatures rose to 106 degrees and caused a condition called disseminated intravascular coagulation that led to liver and kidney failure. We suspect the unfortunate victims were especially vulnerable to very high body temperatures in this context.

"In our study, we observed mild body temperature elevations in subjects who rested comfortably in bed during the session and were encouraged to drink fluids. Temperature regulation seems to be an area of relative risk associated with MDMA use that can be minimized with attention to the setting, activity levels and hydration status.

"We want to conduct more Phase 1 research into physiological responses—particularly central nervous system function—and safety parameters, and we'd like to extend our research into Phase 2 investigations of MDMA for treating certain patient populations. Initially we'll seek permission to work with end-stage cancer patients whose depression and physiological pain haven't responded to conventional treatments.

"We want to work with this group because accepted medical-psychiatric approaches often don't help them, and because encouraging reports from the 1960s and early 1970s describe the successful use of psychedelics under controlled conditions to reduce pain and suffering in terminal cancer patients, and anecdotal case reports from the 1980s about MDMA and laboratory studies of MDMA's effects on pain threshold.

"Some of the most compelling case reports about MDMA come from New Mexico psychiatrist George Greer. One case that intrigued us was a man who had multiple myeloma with skeletal lesions and severe bone pain that hadn't responded to conventional treatments. Dr. Greer treated the man over 9 months with three MDMA sessions, dramatically reducing his pain and the need for narcotics, and improving his mood. That's an example of how MDMA could be used in treatment. Other interesting research shows that MDMA can increase pain threshold and help morphine reduce pain in lab animals.

"We'd also like permission to evaluate how MDMA may be used to treat other conditions, particularly those—like drug and alcohol abuse and chronic post-traumatic stress disorder—that respond poorly to conventional treatments. The treatment model for clinical research [with hallucinogens] would be quite unlike conventional psychiatric therapies. The psychoactive agent, in this case MDMA, would be used to augment the psychotherapy sessions and not just relieve target symptoms.

"I do have concerns about MDMA, particularly for people with underlying vulnerabilities, who use a great deal of it and take it under circumstances that increase the risks. But the neurotoxicity question is controversial. Given our current knowledge of MDMA, it has yet to be rigorously established that MDMA is neurotoxic in humans. And it hasn't been established that MDMA actually damages brain function in animals. Even when lab animals get repeated megadoses of MDMA—much more than a standard human dose—that seem to destroy serotonergic axons [neurons that transport serotonin], no one has shown that this changes behavior in the animals. Also, most MDMA-induced serotonergic degeneration is short term, and lots of the neurons regenerate.

"A related issue worth considering is the case of fenfluramine, a popular federally approved medication used for weight control. Fenfluramine and MDMA cause virtually identical serotonergic axonal degeneration in the brains of lab animals. But fenfluramine's been given over 30 years to 25 million people worldwide with no reports of drug-induced neurotoxicity. In people who've taken MDMA there's also a surprising lack of evidence of a clinical neurotoxicity syndrome. Isolated reports of psychopathology and neurologic injury have been published—particularly in people who take lots of different drugs including large repeated doses of MDMA—there's no apparent pattern of clinical neural degeneration syndromes reported in millions of people who've taken MDMA over the last 20 years.

"The findings of lab research in animals is of genuine concern, but indications now are that it's not so significant when considering a potential treatment in patients with severe clinical disorders that don't respond to conventional therapies and who would take MDMA a few times under very controlled conditions. When assessing the relative merits of any drug, one must always examine the balance between treatment risks and benefits.

"My greater concern is with people who take repeated high doses of MDMA, often with alcohol and other drugs and under adverse conditions. Young people may be at particular risk because they don't completely understand the drug's effects and may tend to act impulsively and with a relative disregard for personal safety. Others at risk are people who take stimulant drugs or monoamine oxidase inhibitor (MAOI) antidepressants, and people with heart conditions. People who take MDMA often and at high doses are likely to be at greatest risk.

"For people who take [MDMA] every week and stack dosages—particularly those who may be sitting on a lot of vulnerability for psychopathology—I'm concerned about the long-term effects. That's what you found in the '60s. People who became long-term psychotics after taking LSD were pretty much ready to take that dive anyway. And the LSD trip hurled them off the edge.

"An ancient Greek axiom of pharmacology says the difference between a medicine and a poison is the dose. As with many accepted and valuable medicines, this may be the case with MDMA."

RICHARD GLENNON ON MDMA

Professor of medicinal chemistry, Department of Medicinal Chemistry, Medical College of Virginia School of Pharmacy, Virginia Commonwealth University, Richmond.

"MDMA is toxic—it destroys certain neurons in the brain, mostly serotonin neurons—but nobody really knows what that means long-term. It's toxic but so's amphetamine, which has been around for 50 years. I'm not saying it should be ignored, I'm saying I don't know what that means. [One researcher] said it was like administering time bombs to people and not knowing when or if they were going to go off. So, 20 years down the road, people who took MDMA or many of these other compounds could have all kinds of neurological deficits. Nobody really has any idea."

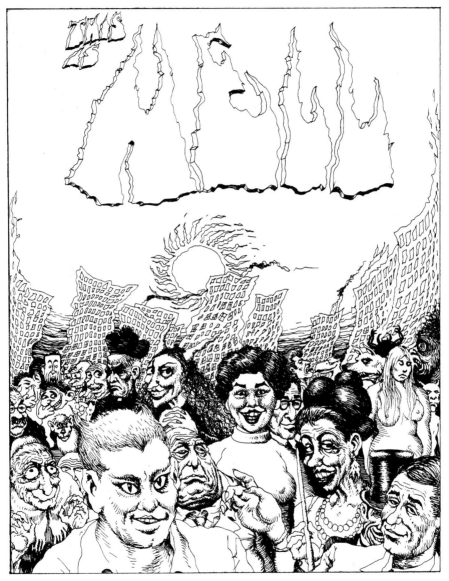

MEMORIES OF A HEAVY LSD TRIP
RECORDED IN THE SKETCHBOOK A FEW
DAYS LATER ~ SAN FRANCISCO, SPRING, '67

DOONESBURY

By G.B. Trudeau

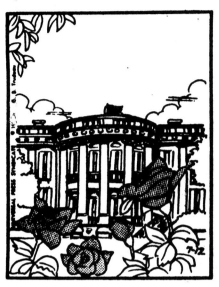

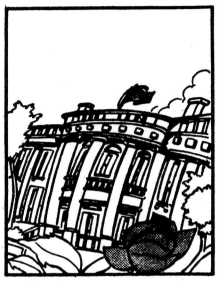

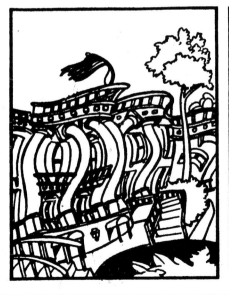

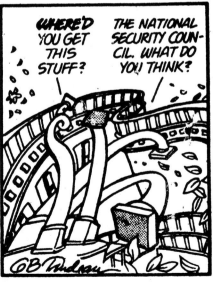

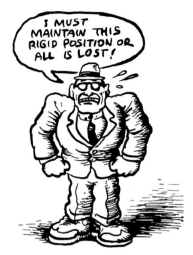

Chapter 10

GATEKEEPERS: YOUR GOVERNMENT ON DRUGS

DEA, FDA, NIDA: Two of these federal agencies regulate hallucinogens. The Drug Enforcement Administration (DEA) has the power to giveth and taketh away—from physicians, pharmacies and researchers—licenses to buy, sell and work with controlled substances like hallucinogens. The Food and Drug Administration (FDA) handles drug safety (they won't kill you) and efficacy (they do exactly what the developers say they'll do) and evaluates applications from people who want to develop new drugs. The National Institute on Drug Abuse (NIDA) funds basic research that promotes its antidrug-abuse mission.

Three people who stay up to their eyebrows most days with the issues of regulating and funding hallucinogen research are Gene Haislip, deputy assistant administrator and director of the Office of Diversion Control for DEA; Curtis Wright, M.D., deputy director of the Division of Anaesthetic, Critical Care and Addiction Drugs and team leader for addiction products at FDA; and Dr. Geraline Lin in the Division of Basic

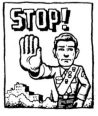

Research at NIDA. Here's where they stand on drug control, hallucinogens, humans as research subjects in hallucinogen studies, people who use street drugs, and the '60s, the '90s and beyond. It's not always what you expect.

DRUG ENFORCEMENT ADMINISTRATION (DEA)

From an August 1996 interview with Gene Haislip, deputy assistant administrator and director of the Office of Diversion Control, Drug Enforcement Administration, U.S. Department of Justice.

"[The DEA controls drugs through] five schedules. Of the five, Schedules II through IV deal with drugs that have legitimate medical purposes. Schedule I is reserved for substances that don't have an approved medical use. If you examine the structure of the law, you see these schedules have graduated degrees of control. The maximum requirements are for Schedule I. The whole purpose of drug scheduling is to recognize two important differences in applying the law to drugs and substances. The first is the relative abuse liability and risk involved with the drug. The second is legitimate society's relative need for availability.

"Take a drug like morphine. It's extremely addictive and potent—a very dangerous drug. Nevertheless, it has a legitimate purpose and there's a limited need for availability—the only time you use morphine is in very serious medical procedures. It's much more limited than drugs like codeine tablets, which you might have to take if you go to the dentist. Codeine is much more generally needed and also happens to be less potent. So codeine is in Schedule III, morphine ends up in Schedule II.

"Schedule I is reserved for substances for which there's an extremely limited need for availability. In fact, the only need for availability is research. So under the law one is justified in putting it in the most restricted category. A lot of substances are in that category. Heroin, for example, one of the most potent narcotics circulating in the U.S. And marijuana, considerably less potent than heroin. And all the substances in between. What Schedule I substances have in common is an extremely limited need for legitimate availability. That need is scientific research. The maximum requirements and some very high penalties exist on that schedule because the only uses we've seen for Schedule I drugs, with the exception of research, are abuse and trafficking.

"We register about 900,000 professionals and business entities to engage in various activities regarding these substances and schedules. Of the 900,000, almost all are physicians. Pharmacies make up another large piece, then manufacturers, wholesale distributors and others. Within that figure are people who apply to us to conduct research on Schedule I substances. Between 900 and 1,000 people, institutions or both are registered at any given time to do research on Schedule I drugs. They have to submit an application to DEA, plus a protocol explaining the drug they want to study and for what purpose.

"Then we start a background investigation to make sure the applicant doesn't have a police record or a reputation for engaging in drug violations, that he or she hasn't lost a previous drug registration, that they're licensed by the state to practice their profession, that they have a premises and the facilities to maintain proper physical security over the substance, that they know how to handle the substance, and they can maintain the required records. That usually won't take more than six weeks. At the same time we send the protocol to the Department of Health and Human Services [DHHS] so they can confirm it's legitimate. That process varies but normally takes something like six weeks. We find the actual response from DHHS varies. It will be relatively brief or it could take much longer. In some cases it's taken a number of months. We've had complaints about that. On one occasion it took a year. We [looked into it and] discovered [DHHS] hadn't done their thing. That's the process we use. And each of the 1,000 who study Schedule I drugs is registered for one or more specific substances in that schedule. The registration is renewable; they need a new one every year."

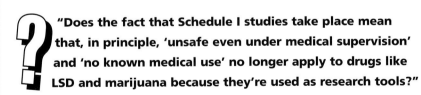

"Does the fact that Schedule I studies take place mean that, in principle, 'unsafe even under medical supervision' and 'no known medical use' no longer apply to drugs like LSD and marijuana because they're used as research tools?"

"There's no approved medical use for marijuana [as there is for synthetic THC, marijuana's main psychoactive ingredient]. The only people legally using it are registered under research protocols or associated with the research—maybe 12 people in the U.S. All substances that might become drugs *do* have to be studied, and eventually in humans, before they're approved. For example, marijuana contains more than and 400 chemicals, of which approximately 60 are called cannabinoids. Delta-9THC is thought to be the primary psychoactive substance in marijuana. THC was singled out for investigation to treat nausea problems. THC was investigated through research on humans before it was approved as a medicine. So there was a time in there when human beings were consuming [THC], not pursuant to a lawful prescription but to lawful research. And [the research] could have gone either way.

"Based on research results, THC could have been discarded as useless [instead of being approved as a medication]. And it's a fairly lengthy period as a rule. The first thing you do is a chemistry study, then experiment with the substance in some animals and eventually in primates and, if everything is still going along, human beings. But that's all research for a substance that has no established medical use. THC moved through that cycle, now doctors can write prescriptions for synthetic THC. That's legal, and we set a production quota for the year based on THC's prescribing history."

"The marijuana plant itself has lots of components that haven't been quantified like THC has. Is that why the whole marijuana plant can't be used medically but THC can?"

"There are other reasons, too. That's just one of them. [When people smoke marijuana,] there's really no way to control the dose. Every marijuana preparation has a different degree of activity. There's no way to standardize the dose. Conceivably you *could* [measure the dose first, then label it somehow], but it's not been done. Plus the other molecules and the tars [haven't been quantified]."

"Cigarettes are legal and they have tars."

"Wait a minute. We don't judge drug policy based on cigarettes or alcohol because the law specifically says we can't control them. I'm sure it's obvious that they meet the scheduling criteria and would be controlled otherwise. But Congress says we can't do that—for historical reasons, I presume."

"Some Schedule I drugs are no different [in terms of addiction and toxicity] than alcohol and cigarettes."

"They're all different but they all create their own problems. In theory, any of these drugs could be developed for a medical purpose."

"These are drugs people tend to abuse, but researchers are the ones who suffer. Scheduling tends to make it harder for researchers to get Schedule I drugs—LSD for example—to study, to figure out why they're abused, to understand why some are seen as public health problems."

"I'd have to disagree. You have to understand that all the drugs in all the schedules are abused. Codeine, heroin, marijuana. They're all abused and there are registration requirements for everyone, except patients, who handle them. There are no such requirements for patients, just as there are no such requirements for research subjects. If you're a doctor prescribing any of these drugs, you have to register. A researcher has to register, too. Researchers *do* register and there is no impediment. The only impediments are self-imposed. If researchers don't have the money or the interest or the sponsorship, *then* they have a problem. But under the law they have no particular problem. They can apply for registration and about 1,000 do. We've turned down very few who apply. They have requirements to meet but so does every physician, every pharmacist, every manufacturer, for products in the other four Schedules. So I don't feel [researchers are unduly restricted by Schedule I]. There is *one* problem in engaging in pharmaceutical research—it's expensive. You have to have somebody who can do it or who has the backing to do it, but that's not a problem connected with drug control policy."

"Schedule I has two parts: the drug has no approved medical use and it's highly abusable. Some researchers want DEA to expand Schedule I to include a Schedule I-a just for researchers that acknowledges the dangers, leaves the restrictions in place, but makes the drugs more available for research and treatment by those who have special training—like complicated surgical procedures that only certain surgeons with certain training can do at certain centers with appropriate monitoring, safeguards and supervision."

"But that *is* the purpose of Schedule I. It was designed for them."

"It's not working. I hate to be the one to tell you this."

"It's certainly working fine from our point of view because there's no difficulty in registering people. It doesn't take a great deal of time and very seldom do we disapprove anyone who seeks to register. If there are problems, they have nothing to do with applying the law. What they may be concerned with is the so-called orphan drug problem, which is the difficulty of obtaining financial backing for some types of research. We have registered people for research on these drugs since the law's been in force—since 1970. But we don't influence funding."

"Maybe the drugs' Schedule I status gives them a negative image among potential funding agencies or institutions."

"I think what you're not seeing is that it frequently takes time and money to develop pharmaceuticals. A lot of pharmaceuticals are developed; quite a few aren't. When they aren't, sometimes it's because the pharmaceutical industry isn't interested. Most money to develop pharmaceuticals comes from the pharmaceutical industry, based on their evaluation of the substance's potential. It has nothing to do with DEA law or FDA law. The law is designed to make sure a drug is sufficiently researched before it's used in medicine. That's what the laws require to protect the public. You wouldn't want your doctor prescribing a medication that hadn't been researched for safety and efficacy. This is the protection the law requires. But which drugs are selected for development and how they're developed aren't involved in applying these laws. Some programs in funding agencies sometimes assist development, as was the case in AIDS and has been the case occasionally in cancer. But DEA and FDA are not funding agencies. Those problems are of a different nature. We don't get involved in them at all.

"Someone felt THC was worth spending money on. And they developed it and got approval for it. That's a case where it's been done. Theoretically, it can be done in any of these cases. It's a question of utility. At this point, none of the other drugs seems to have shown enough utility to entice someone to go further with it. If research shows [a drug's] value, then it could be approved. Let's take [LSD psychotherapy] as an example. Suppose research established some medical use for LSD. Then it could be approved. Researchers would have to do a study, then go through FDA's Investigative New Drug [IND] process. They can do it but they have to go through the process. Anyone who has the interest and believes in the possibility can explore that. Of course, they must have the [appropriate scientific] credentials."

"Might a Schedule I listing discourage interest from potential funding institutions?"

"That may be. There's nothing one can do about that. A lot of problems come about because of peoples' abuses. It may have a [negative] effect but that doesn't eliminate the need for research. There's research on alcoholism and that has a lot of associated problems. There's no choice because the substances have problems and have to be controlled. If that creates a stigma, that's unfortunate. But a number of drugs have gone through this development process. If they can be developed, they should be because all the drugs in Schedules II through IV are abused, some of them very heavily. In fact, more than half the top 20 drugs of abuse are legitimate drugs—they're not even in Schedule I. One can look in the other categories and see the same problems. The point is that if a substance is shown to have a legitimate value, it will be approved and made available even though there are abuse problems connected with it. And many are."

"Doesn't the fact that there's an abuse problem automatically make Schedule I drugs important research topics—to learn why they're abused, what causes the abuse?"

"That's a different type of research and I certainly think it's very important. But we don't need to modify the schedules because they already provide a technique to [study these questions]. What is *not* our mission is to help get it done, whereas that is the mission of NIDA and other [funding agencies]. We do have a method to permit it and the mechanism works.

"Drugs should be researched and developed for legitimate medical purposes. That's the proper context in which they should be consumed. They should not be consumed for any other purpose. All medicines are dangerous and have to be used with a great deal of caution. A lot of people are injured by legitimate medication because of the way it's prescribed and consumed. It's not only true for controlled drugs, it's true for antibiotics and lots of different drugs. They all have dangers. The object of the system is to minimize the dangers and maximize the medical potential. As to Schedule I drugs, we do know of a case [THC] where that was done. If there are others, I think everybody will welcome it. And there's no impediment."

"Some researchers think the mechanism is too restrictive."

"I don't know how many feel that way, but I would say that's an expression of ignorance on their part—ignorance of the way the laws and requirements work—because it's not really an impediment. The capability is there and we have the record to prove it. There are people who get registered and conduct this research. Those who wish to can, and there's no calendar or anything. You can apply on any day."

 FOOD AND DRUG ADMINISTRATION (FDA)

From a March 1996 personal interview with Curtis Wright, M.D., then deputy director in the FDA Division of Anaesthetic, Critical Care and Addiction Drugs, and team leader for addiction products.

"Let me try to put things in perspective. Through the 1960s and '70s, FDA's role with respect to drugs of abuse was very conservative. FDA was seen as protecting the culture from those who would use the drugs improperly. At that time all protocols involving potential drugs of abuse, including hallucinogens, went through FDA's Drug Abuse Advisory Committee, which determined if the protocol's scientific merit warranted the risk of exposing individuals [in human trials] to the drugs. There were a lot of reasons for that. One was that we genuinely didn't know what the long-term danger from exposure to these agents were. There were some horrific dosing accidents in and around the [1967] Summer of Love. Some nasty, toxic, misbranded products were sold in that period and the result was fear that exposure to hallucinogens would permanently injure people. In that era we described flashbacks as the inevitable consequence of LSD use, and we were very concerned about the effect of intravenous amphetamine abuse on cognition. So there was a tremendous conservatism about allowing research with hallucinogenic compounds except under very careful control. The careful control was that a researcher would write a protocol, bring it to FDA and agency staff would review it and present it at committee meetings that were held once or twice a year. The committee would review the protocol, make suggestions, the individual would go back and implement those suggestions and, in some cases, the research actually went forward. But the process was very onerous and lengthy."

"What happened next?"

"Over time a number of individuals, some inside, some outside government asked, *Should this be the case? Is it appropriate to have such a high level of concern for these agents that we would not have, for example, for a cancer chemotherapy that might prove fatal?* And there was no good answer. We didn't have the same kind of restrictions for the [potentially fatal] cancer chemotherapy. If there was concern about a protocol, you might very well go through the same kind of process. In other words, if you had a new drug and you were genuinely unsure of the protocol's safety, you might take it to the Advisory Committee in closed session and the review might take longer. But the agency was challenged legally in a number of cases and also underwent a process of introspection, asking, *Is it proper to treat this class of drugs differently?* That culminated in 1989 or 1990, when we were fortunate to have the National Institute on Drug Abuse challenge FDA to do a better job in the area of addictions treatment. They used a variety of mechanisms: Senator Edward Kennedy and Senator Joe Biden held hearings in which the senior agency staff was directly pressed—*What are you doing?* So part of the legislation that implemented the NIDA medications development program mandated effective review at FDA. We all got a trip downtown and had a lovely hearing in front of Senator Biden, where we heard some very critical words about what FDA was doing. [As a] consequence, three people were hired [and specifically assigned to drug abuse issues]—myself, Corrine Moody and Mike Klein. The center director put [us] in an experimental unit called Pilot Drug Staff. [Our] mission was to focus on process *outcome* rather than process.

"We were essentially told, *It is far more important that your decisions be in the country's best interest than that they follow the agency's traditional process.* Regulatory agencies have a chronic tension between process and outcome. We're given the process by law—we aren't free to say, *Let's do it different today.* [In 1989-90,] Pilot Drug got specific regulatory permission to depart from traditional agency practices in a number of ways. And we did. Some worked and some didn't. One thing that worked was that we went back through every single Investigative New Drug (IND) application that was still active but on clinical hold. Every single one. And we started calling people. We found requests for hallucinogen research, marijuana research, LSD research, undercapitalized venture-capital drug products—all kinds of things—but many were put on hold and no one had figured out how to break them free.

"In the same way, there's something almost holy or magic about people's brains. The concept of damaging your brain is a horror. And all of these drugs have some animal somewhere that shouldn't take it. Mark Molliver [a hallucinogen researcher at Johns Hopkins University in Baltimore] clearly demonstrated that rats shouldn't take MDMA [ecstasy] or ibogaine. The question we had to wrestle with was: *What does that mean? Should we pass laws restricting rat access to MDMA or DMT or ibogaine? Or should we use it to guide human work?* We found ourselves in some very disturbing situations. At a time when maybe 10 or 20 percent of college students in the country were taking ecstasy, all the IND protocols for research on ecstasy were on clinical hold because [the drug] was perceived as too unsafe even to study.

"Now there's a difference between self-administering a drug and legitimate research, and it's something we have to wrestle with. If a person says, *I will take this [drug] as an illegal act*, and something bad happens to them, that's their problem. If you walk in dressed in a white coat and hand them a capsule of MDMA, and something bad happens to them, that's *your* problem. Because when it comes to biomedical research, our culture—for all its honor and the American mystique of personal freedom—is still very paternalistic. It's the researcher's responsibility. There is the liability and that's real. But, in fact, there have been very few successful suits. Litigation risk is not a real serious concern. What is a serious concern is the feeling of horror on the part of researchers if they injure someone. No one wants to hurt a research volunteer.

"The conclusion was that the Food and Drug Administration was going to treat all drugs the same. All drugs have risks, all have benefits. All drug research has risks, all drug research has benefits. This policy actually represents no change because that's what we were always supposed to do. So [in late 1994 or early 1995], the deputy center director wrote a very nice statement. It said basically that we were going to treat [hallucinogens, marijuana, and other drugs of abuse] no differently than any other [drug]. That's what the advisory committee recommended and that's what we've done ever since. Because at that point we'd been through a lot of wrestling over ibogaine, MDMA, LSD—over a whole class of serotonergic drugs [that work at serotonin receptors in the brain] that rats shouldn't take.

"Clearly, some drugs at some doses will change your brain. For many days one has a clue what that means. We're concerned and a little anxious because the same pathways some doses of some drugs permanently affect are also receptors that [antidepressants] like Prozac affect. We're worried about what's going to happen to these people long-term, and we don't know."

 "How can FDA approve a drug like Prozac that works at the same brain receptors as hallucinogens, and not approve hallucinogen research in humans?"

"One appears to be reversible and the other appears not to be—as when an animal model demonstrated that [MDMA, ibogaine and some amphetamines] caused permanent, irreversible change[s in brain neurons]. We have no problem knowing what to do if the animal falls over or goes blind or can't walk. But how do you tell if a rat's judgment is impaired? It's difficult because they can't tell us. So we continue to struggle with [the fact that] many approved drugs cause changes in the central nervous system. Many cancer drugs have neurotoxic effects. But most people, even most physicians, consider risking a little neurotoxicity as opposed to dying to be a reasonable trade. The question ultimately boils down to, *What are you treating and what benefit do you want, versus what are you risking and does that make sense to most of us?* That's where we are.

"There are people on this planet who believe the government has no business whatsoever restricting the pharmaceuticals they wish to take. Others on the planet have an equally firm belief that it's the government's responsibility to protect them from agents that might cause them harm, to the point of restricting several important constitutional freedoms. Both groups come in and talk to the FDA. Often. We end up trying to be a fair judge and arbiter. In the main, we succeed.

"Two issues are involved in regulating hallucinogens. FDA doesn't regulate the practices of medicine or pharmacy, the states do. We regulate the pharmaceutical industry so we regulate the shipment, the interstate traffic of substances for use in biomedical research. We also regulate the function and composition of institutional review boards that must approve research in humans to protect the subjects, to make sure their ethical freedoms are protected. DEA has statutory responsibility for the importation, production, transportation and use of controlled substances, and a very high degree of concern about controlled substances that have no approved medical use. If you want to do research in humans and you need permission, come to FDA. If you need permission to manufacture, ship, handle, possess, transport or dispense a controlled substance, go to DEA.

"States also have jurisdiction over research. For example, California has an independent research board. You have to clear [state and federal boards] so it's potentially a long road for a scientist to do hallucinogen research. That's not a bad thing. If I had to characterize the hallucinogen research situation, I'd say hallucinogen research is not something you can do impulsively. You have to really want to do it and be willing to make a convincing case that it's appropriate. You'll get an opportunity to conduct your research if a potential benefit outweighs the sometimes known and sometimes unknown risks."

"In terms of FDA's inclination to protect people from certain drugs, what's the difference between 1965 and 1996?"

"The culture has changed, and cultural changes affect the government. The Summer of Love occurred when I was in my sophomore year of college and it altered my life. I went through all the cultural changes the '60s brought. I lost innocence that can never be regained with respect to scientific and governmental institutions. All my staff at this point have grown up realizing that government, medical and scientific practitioners can be right or wrong, helpful or destructive. And that we have the responsibility, individually and collectively, to see that it's right and constructive.

"In the 1960s we faced an epidemic and it's wonderful that we had as few casualties as we did. Drug abuse and dependence are horrific, lethal conditions, and it was only in 1994-95 that we began to understand how deadly it is. If you're a multisubstance abuser in America and you live in an urban area, your annual mortality rate can be as high as 5 to 8 percent. That's all-cause mortality—overdosed, medically sick, shot, AIDS. The result is that an epidemic of mortality associated with drug abuse and dependence is the most serious cause of premature death we face. It's clear that a *laissez faire* attitude toward drugs isn't possible. Individuals in the culture get killed by drugs and suffer horribly before they die. By the same token, many [drugs]—as a side effect or as part of therapy or related to therapy—change the function of the brain. But we can't be unwilling to accept them as medicines because they're hallucinogenic, either. If I had to characterize how the agency got to this [perspective]—speaking for reviewers who look at the protocols and make decisions—they recognize that they must always make balanced decisions; be fair and respectful of those who would do things [they wouldn't do]."

"What about the traditional Western notion that people should only take drugs when they're sick?"

"Nobody believes that anymore. People who develop and regulate drugs abandoned that years ago. We have lots of drugs people take to affect their bodies or minds in ways that aren't directly related to changing a disease state. An example is cholesterol-lowering agents. We think if you have high cholesterol, you should have it lowered. If you have an appropriate medicine to make it lower and reduce your risk of heart attack, that's a good thing."

"What about less tangible things like expanding consciousness or having mystical experiences?"

If someone believes an ibogaine experience or an MDMA experience may help someone deal with drug dependency or the pain of cancer or the emotional pain of their lives or work more effectively in therapy—those things can be measured. FDA doesn't deal with recreational drug use. We genuinely are committed to our mission of health and quality of life. Pharmacology as recreation is someone else's concern. Like those who have to deal with alcohol-containing beverages. Those sorts of things generally are managed at the state level. We *become* concerned when somebody's recreational activity becomes somebody else's terminal event.

"[Looking toward the future,] most of the easy parts of neurochemistry we know about. We have agents that alter neurochemistry in rather crude ways right now, and there's subtlety with respect to the brain that we don't know a lot about. I think a great deal of important, positive things will happen, some of which will involve the neural pathways associated with hallucinogenic phenomena. They clearly do something in the brain; they're clearly important in the brain. What they do and why they're important is something people are actively pursuing. I'm very optimistic. Something good will come from this but it will be a long, hard struggle because we design our rules and laws for two groups in our culture—the most virtuous and the least virtuous. Part of the job of good government is to assure the laws passed to deal with people who are genuine predators—and they exist—don't inhibit the rest of the population. That's our continuing challenge."

 "Does it make sense that at one time 10-20 percent of college students were taking a drug [ecstasy] the FDA considered too dangerous to study?"

"No, it doesn't make sense. The committee said it didn't make sense and I don't think we'll find ourselves in that situation again. There's a genuine emerging recognition of the rights of the rest of us. That's probably part of the future—the notion that the rest of us have rights too. You have advocates and proponents; they're vocal and hold extreme positions. And you have people who think the advocates are terrible; they hold another extreme position. The rest of us are in the middle but we have rights. When the sons and daughters of Americans are exposed to a drug that may hurt them for life, it's incumbent on the scientific community to try to find out the truth and to act reasonably."

 NATIONAL INSTITUTE ON DRUG ABUSE (NIDA)

 From a March 1996 personal interview with Dr. Geraline Lin, program officer, Division of Basic Research at the National Institute on Drug Abuse in Bethesda, Maryland.

"[NIDA] has many focuses but our primary goal is to try to take care of drug abuse problems—all kinds of substance abuse. When you do that kind of research, you inevitably link into public health and all kinds of health-related issues. For instance, in the case of hallucinogen research, [hallucinogens] have been abused and that's a problem. We want to be able to take care of the problem. But while we are doing research on that, it's inevitable we will touch the area of how hallucinogens work in the brain. We know in a way how our mental processes and mental states are exhibited—how the mechanism works—and that [LSD] causes a tremendous change in mental state. If we know the underlying mechanism, we'll have knowledge about how to deal with the problem and we'll know a lot more about brain activities associated with mental health. Our primary interest is solving the drug abuse problem, but if we can reveal this underlying fundamental process, that will have a very big impact on understanding mental activity and mental health. It's not all strictly related to drug abuse, but it's hard to separate those things. When you take [LSD], your mental status shifts. What's going on in the brain? What processes of information integration underlie all that? What triggers the manifestation of the changing mental state? The impact is beyond anything I can think of. We do have a lot of information and funding compared to 10 or 15 years ago.

"The problem is, [hallucinogen research on humans] has been banned for almost 30 years. But during that time we continued animal research and made tremendous progress in studying this class of drug in animals. The brain is complex, but compared to 30 years ago we know so much more—about 5-HT and the 5-HT [family of] receptors and other systems. In the 1960s, people just used [LSD] and described what happened. I don't mean that kind of information isn't useful. But it's also necessary to have scientific information, well-controlled and gathered by [credentialed] investigators."

"In the 1960s when psychedelics were banned as dangerous, federal officials who lowered the boom must not have known enough about LSD to characterize it as dangerous."

"Obviously if there are problems with a drug, the chances of exposing it rises with the number of people who use it. If the magnitude is such that federal officials are alerted and become concerned about public health, I would imagine they'd feel a need to take some action. That would probably be the case even if they didn't know the exact problem. That's my interpretation."

"I'd think research efforts would be more aggressive for a drug that was so mysterious, powerful and taken by so many people."

"Yes and no. [LSD] has the ability to produce such a profound effect that you know more about its implications than anything else. It touches everyone's life, it's really profound—that's what makes it so interesting. On the other hand, you know that people abuse it and want to get high and some have problems. Whether the problems are ascribed to the right thing or not, people still have the same kinds of problems over and over. That's definitely a public health concern. You're talking about a balance between interest in

HIGHLIGHTS: NIDA-FUNDED HALLUCINOGEN RESEARCH
Human Research

PRINCIPAL INVESTIGATOR & RESEARCH	PROJECT PERIOD

George Ricaurte, Neurology
Johns Hopkins University, Baltimore, Maryland

Research 1: Define the health consequences of MDMA use and explain serotonin's role in the central nervous system.	March 1, 1994– February 28, 1999
Research 2: Study recreational MDMA users to document damage to serotonin neurons in the brain.	August 1, 1991– February 28, 2000
Research 3: Validate the utility of a compound called MCN to detect drug-induced serotonin neurotoxicity, and use it with positron emission tomography (PET) scan imaging to assess serotonin system damage in people with MDMA abuse histories.	September 30, 1995– August 31, 1998

RICK STRASSMAN, Psychiatry
University of New Mexico, Albuquerque

Research: Describe how DMT exerts its biological and psychological effects.	March 1, 1993– June 30, 1996

HENRY HOLCOMB, Psychiatry
University of Maryland, Baltimore

Research: Define the functional neuroanatomy of ketamine-induced psychosis.	September 30, 1994– August 31, 1997

DAVID OSTROW, Psychiatry and Behavioral Medicine
Medical College of Wisconsin, Milwaukee

Research: Develop and evaluate a behavioral cognitive skills development approach to reducing risky behavior in gay and bisexual men who recreationally use marijuana, hallucinogens and other drugs.	July 15, 1995– May 31, 1999

FRANCESCO CHIAPPELLI, Anatomy and Cell Biology
University of California, Los Angeles

Research: Conduct *in vitro* experiments to test the effects of cocaine and PCP on CD4 lymphocyte [white blood cell] function, maturation and molecular processes.	August 15, 1992– June 30, 1997

[LSD] and the possibility that it might cause problems. In the '60s many people were exposed and all the reports say there were many problems. That's what caused a ban [on research] and DEA was made responsible for controlling it. That's why everything was put on hold. If you're a public official, you can't ignore a public health problem. Someone has to make a decision, analyze the risks and benefits. Even though human studies were banned, [NIDA] always had animal studies going."

"Why, after all those years, did NIDA decide to fund Rick Strassman's DMT study on human volunteers in 1991?"

"Because until that point we simply couldn't do human studies. To get to the approval stage for human studies, [Dr. Strassman] had to go through a lot of hurdles with FDA. It took him a couple of years to get that [approval]. Most people feel it's too much trouble to go through when they can't even be sure they'll win the battle.

"To do *human* studies, [researchers] have to go through FDA and DEA. All new drugs have to go through the IND [Investigative New Drug] approval process. Then, if they work with a controlled substance, they have to go through DEA. If FDA doesn't approve [the protocol for human trials], we can't fund the project. [NIDA] can't fund any project that's not approved by FDA. But we can help grantees with protocols before they go through review process. Our job is to help grantees. That's no problem. LSD is Schedule I so [hallucinogen researchers] have to deal with DEA, and they want to do human studies so they have to deal with FDA. On top of that, the 1960s gave LSD a notorious reputation. A lot of people, for instance pharmaceutical companies, simply don't want to touch this area. It's taboo!

"On our part, I don't feel [NIDA's] guilty of anything. We promote [hallucinogen studies] because we see the importance of the research. Our primary interest is to solve the drug-abuse problem and we want to know how to take care of problems [related to] hallucinogens. But if we study a powerful drug like LSD and learn something that's a breakthrough in [brain research], I don't think we'd mind taking credit for unraveling how LSD works and changes mental activity and affects mental health.

"Unfortunately, [in designing studies and developing research protocols for hallucinogens,] a lot of researchers try to use short cuts. That's not good. If they used the same kind of rigid, well-designed studies investigators use for other kinds of drugs, they would be in a position to convince other scientists. If they don't, they will always have doubters, people with reservations [who will never fully support them]. The best way is to deal with it head on, go to a credible kind of protocol evaluation and firmly establish the drug's credibility. Researchers may try to take short cuts because mental activity is hard to measure, so they think they shouldn't have to go through all those processes. Studies on stomach aches or chronic pain are easier to measure, more objective. But here we're talking about mental state—they need to design technologies to measure it. This is more complicated, admittedly. They need to identify [the question], say what the research is all about and find some way to answer the question. With new methodology and new technology, I'm sure they will find a way to study [hallucinogens]. People need proof, and we start with peer review to evaluate the scientific merit. We want to do it the proper way. If there's something to [the research], we can establish that. If hallucinogen researchers can't [go through the process], they'll never get the opportunity to find out one way or the other [if hallucinogens are worth studying]."

"What's the future of hallucinogen research at NIDA?"

"Animal studies, definitely. In the past we had very little information. Now we have many different animal models. We can do studies at the cellular and molecular levels, and use computer modeling [to fill the gaps]. It's growing in all directions and, on top of that, there's an acute need for human data to validate the animal data. That doesn't mean you just plug the drug into the human. You need to use a proper well-designed control, be a well-qualified, experienced investigator and go through the IND process. Right now there is very little human data. That makes it difficult, but we're doing more and more [human studies]. We've made a lot of progress, yet we still have a long way to go."

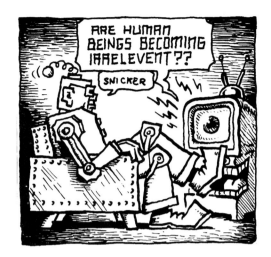

Chapter 11

HALLUCINOGEN RESEARCH INTO THE 21ST CENTURY

"A long way lies ahead in creating and disseminating information through research and education before intelligent decisions can be assured at the individual level."
—Stephen Szára, M.D., D.Sc., 1968

IF RESEARCHERS HAVE learned anything since LSD's development in 1943, it's that the federal government—at least where funding for human hallucinogen studies is concerned—doesn't have its tray table in a fully upright and locked position. In the shiny new 21st century, organizations like the Multidisciplinary Association for Psychedelic Studies (MAPS), the Heffter Research Institute and the Albert Hofmann Foundation will promote, coordinate and help fund hallucinogen research that's free of federal funding's historically negative biases.

 **MAPS**

Multidisciplinary Association For Psychedelic Studies

2121 Commonwealth Dr, Ste 220, ., Charlotte, NC 28205 Tel 704/334.1798 Fax

704/334.1799 **http://www.maps.org**

 MAPS is an IRS-approved 501 (c)(3) nonprofit corporation funded by tax deductible donations from about 1,350 members and chartered in 1986 as a membership-based research and education organization. It mainly works to help psychedelic researchers around the world design, get government approval for, fund, conduct and report on psychedelic research in humans. MAPS publishes a quarterly newsletter for members, government policy makers and academic experts.

One of MAPS' recent efforts has involved working (like a dog) for federal approval to use marijuana as an experimental treatment for conditions like cancer (alleviates chemotherapy's nausea, vomiting and appetite loss); glaucoma (reduces pressure in the eye); multiple sclerosis (reduces muscle pain and spasticity); epilepsy (prevents epileptic seizures in some patients); and chronic pain. In early 1998, the MAPS-sponsored medical marijuana research project, to be conducted by Dr. Donald Abrams, University of California at San Francisco, nearly $1 million from the National Institute on Drug Abuse (NIDA). It'll be the first study of the medical use of marijuana in a patient population in 15 years.

MAPS' founder and president Rick Doblin is in the Ph.D. program in Public Policy at Harvard's Kennedy School of Government. In a June 1996 telephone interview, he said he formed MAPS to "convince Gene Haislip (the deputy assistant administrator, Drug Enforcement Administration) that certain psychedelic drugs deserve to be prescription medicines" and to help make that so by working within the system's bureaucracies, policies and procedures to fund research and deal with political obstacles and diversion control (DEA) issues.

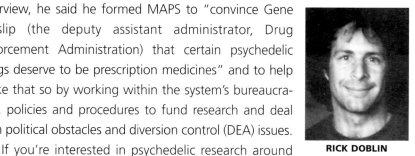

RICK DOBLIN

If you're interested in psychedelic research around the world, offered with no agenda except to fund as much research as possible and distribute the results, MAPS' Web site (**http://www.maps.org**) offers free access to past newsletters, searchable by keyword.

THE HEFFTER RESEARCH INSTITUTE (HRI)

David Nichols, president; HRI, 7 Avenida Vista Grande, Suite B7, Santa Fe, NM 87505

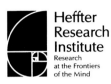
Heffter Research Institute
Research at the Frontiers of the Mind

http://www.heffter.org

The Heffter Research Institute (HRI) was incorporated in New Mexico in 1993 as a nonprofit, 501(c)(3) organization. It's named after Dr. Arthur Heffter, a turn-of-the-century German research pharmacologist who discovered that mescaline was the peyote cactus's main psychoactive element. HRI's position is that psychedelic agents used in well-designed, carefully conducted scientific experiments can be used to further understanding of the mind.

Because psychedelic agents are like natural compounds in the brain, studying their effects on brain function and experiences gives researchers access to primary states of brain and mind and their connections, and an unparalleled chance to understand the relationship between brain and mind. Hallucinogens are an essential technology for investigating chemical, neurological, psychological and spiritual realms in the brain.

HRI funding goes to support research projects at universities and research institutions; collaborate with medical schools and other research institutions to implement specific research efforts and minimize operating costs; develop a credible presence in medical school psychiatry, pharmacology and neuroscience departments; and create a formal program that allows training in scientific and therapeutic uses of psychedelic drugs in the medical community.

CURRENT RESEARCH @ HRI

CLINICAL RESEARCH

MDMA, pain, and psychological distress in terminal cancer patients. Investigators: Charles Grob, M.D., and Russell Poland, Ph.D., Los Angeles, California.

MDMA-assisted psychotherapy may help end-stage cancer patients who don't respond to conventional treatments for chronic physical pain and psychological distress. Psychedelic investigations in cancer patients started in the early 1960s, showing that low-dose LSD could reduce chronic intractable pain associated with disease. It measurably reduced reported pain and the need for narcotics, and patients had less anxiety about and fear of dying. The investigators will study the effects of MDMA treatment in people with end-stage cancers who haven't responded to other pain- and distress-control interventions. Annual cost: $30,000.

The relationship between peak experience and outcome in LSD psychotherapy with substance abusers. Investigators: Albert Kurland, M.D., Richard Yensen, Ph.D., and Donna Dryer, M.D.-M.P.H, Baltimore, Maryland.

This FDA-approved study assesses the effect of different LSD doses on short-term intensive outpatient LSD therapy for drug abusers. The results should give valuable information about predictive factors for positive outcome. The goal is to determine relationships between peak experience as an objectively measured event in LSD psychotherapy, the number of exposures to LSD during psychotherapy and clinical improvement as objective measures of therapeutic outcome. Estimated annual cost: $100,000.

Ecstasy and the brain. Investigators: Alex Gamma and Franz Vollenweider, M.D., Zurich, Switzerland.

Animal studies show that high or repeated doses of MDMA are toxic to certain brain cells. It's unclear whether MDMA is neurotoxic in humans, since average human doses are lower than those used in most animal experiments. This project will shed more light on this question. The Swiss government approved and initially supported the project, but the researchers need more funding to complete it. Annual cost: $30,000.

Ecstasy, psychobiology, and people. Investigators: Charles Grob, M.D., and Russell Poland, Ph.D., Los Angeles, California.

Since May 1994, an FDA-approved Phase I investigation of MDMA's physiological and psychological effects and safety parameters has taken place at the Harbor-UCLA Medical Center. To date, 18 subjects with histories of MDMA use have received MDMA in a double-blind, placebo-controlled model. The most intriguing preliminary finding is elevated cerebral blood flow in subjects with histories of significant MDMA use. In this next investigation of MDMA effects on serotonergic function, 10 subjects and 10 matched normal controls will have brain imaging after taking MDMA; and

10 subjects will enroll in a double-blind, crossover neuroendocrine challenge study to explore serotonergic mechanisms through receptor blockade. Annual cost: $30,000.

Hallucinogens, entactogens, and psychostimulants. Investigators: Euphrosyne Gouzoulis-Mayfrank, M.D., Aachen, Germany, and Mark Geyer, Ph.D., La Jolla, California.

Ecstasy and related drugs are legally hallucinogens, but anecdotal human reports and animal studies suggest their subjective effects and mechanisms of action differ from classical hallucinogens. They may be prototypes of a new class of drugs called entactogens. Most evidence for their distinctive nature comes from animal studies, but Dr. Gouzoulis-Mayfrank published preliminary studies in humans. The investigators want to extend her work in studies of healthy volunteers to compare the effects of a traditional psychostimulant (methamphetamine), a classical hallucinogen (psilocybin) and an entactogen (MDE, Eve) using psychological and neurobiological tests. These will establish differences and similarities among the drugs and examine their mechanisms and sites of action. This study began in 1995 after two years of work to develop protocols, get permissions and find initial support. Cost: $40,000.

Receptor mechanisms and psychedelic drug effects. Investigators: Franz Vollenweider, M.D., Zurich, and Mark Geyer, Ph.D., La Jolla, California.

Different brain neurotransmitter systems may mediate the effects of psychedelics like psilocybin and ketamine. Psilocybin and other classical hallucinogens are thought to act as agonists for the neurotransmitter serotonin; ketamine, phencyclidine and other dissociative anesthetics seem to interact with excitatory amino acid receptors in the brain. But these suggested mechanisms have not been tested in human subjects. This project will combine state-of-the-art psychological, brain imaging and psychophysiological methods to explore sites and mechanisms of action of psilocybin and ketamine in humans. The experimental protocols are approved and some parts of the project are under way, but the work can't be completed without more funding. Cost: $35,000.

ETHNOPHARMACOLOGICAL RESEARCH

Impact of peyotism in the Native American church. Investigators: Neal Goldsmith, Ph.D., New York, and Stacy Schaefer, Ph.D., Edinburg, Texas.

Anecdotal accounts and recent qualitative studies show positive effects of peyotism on mental, physical and social well-being. Decades of literature report a positive impact of peyotism on alcoholism, though there's no research with control groups. Despite such reports, there's no scientific consensus on peyotism's safety and benefits. The goal is to learn about the real-world effects of Native American Church (NAC) peyotism. The researchers will triangulate with multiple methods, including archival research, field research, a mail survey of senior NAC representatives and federal officials and a conference to present findings to NAC participants, study sponsors and the scientific community. Cost: $30,000 (excluding conference).

The chemistry and pharmacology of psychoactive mint. Investigators: Dennis McKenna, Ph.D., Minneapolis, Minnesota, and Deborah Mash, Ph.D., Miami, Florida.

Salvia divinorum is a psychoactive member of the mint family (*Labiatae*) used in shamanic rituals by the Mazatecs and other indigenous people of the Mexican highlands. Ethnobotanical and archeological data show the divinatory use of *Salvia divinorum* is ancient. Recent chemical and pharmacological investigations isolated a new class of potent psychoactive substances, and preliminary screening of the compounds against major classes of neurotransmitter receptors show that previously uncharacterized receptors in the central nervous system may mediate their effects. Pilot projects seek to isolate enough Salvinorin A from *Salvia divinorum* for pharmacological studies; characterize the pharmacological properties of Salvinorin A; and isolate and characterize related compounds from one or more related *Salvia* species. Cost: $30,000.

The human psychopharmacology of ayahuasca—Phase II. Investigators: Dennis McKenna, Ph.D., Minneapolis, Minnesota, and Charles Grob, M.D., Los Angeles, California.

The Hoasca (same as ayahuasca) Project is an interdisciplinary biomedical investigation in humans of acute and long-term effects of ayahuasca, a psychedelic beverage prepared from Amazonian plants and consumed by members of the Uniao do Vegetal (UDV), a Brazilian syncretic sect, in collective rituals. The Hoasca Project began in 1993. The initial study sought to accumulate baseline data on acute and long-term psychological and physiological effects of regular hoasca ingestion in humans. Data collected so far contains unexpected, potentially significant results and suggests directions for future research. Funding is needed for follow-up studies and to expand previous work. Cost: $30,000-$200,000.

Ethnopharmacologic search for psychoactive drugs II. Conference Organizer: Dennis McKenna, Ph.D., Minneapolis, Minnesota.

In 1967, a landmark conference on the history of psychedelics was held in San Francisco under the sponsorship of what was then the Department of Health, Education and Welfare (DHEW). The invitational conference was called the Ethnopharmacologic Search for Psychoactive Drugs. Research in the field continues and researchers have made new discoveries. The conference organizers want to hold a second conference in 1997, *Ethnopharmacologic Search for Psychoactive Drugs II: 30 Years Later*. Cost: $50,000-$80,000. The Heffter Institute has commitments of up to $25,000; the organizers seek matching donations.

PRECLINICAL RESEARCH

Receptor profiles of LSD-related lysergamides. Investigator: David Nichols, Ph.D., West Lafayette, Indiana.

Psychedelic agents can be divided into phenethylamines (related to mescaline) and tryptamines. LSD is a special example of a tryptamine. Pharmacological studies show that phenethylamine-type agents seem to bind tightly to two types of brain serotonin receptors. Tryptamines bind to a third serotonin receptor type, while LSD binds to several more serotonin receptor types, alpha adrenergic receptors and at least two dopamine receptor types. Since LSD is the most potent psychedelic agent, its effects may relate to this multireceptor binding. Early clinical studies with lysergamides like LSD found them less potent than LSD. This project would develop receptor binding profiles for lysergamides that have been tested in humans to correlate pharmacological effects with an affinity for certain receptors. Estimated cost: $30,000.

◤ THE ALBERT HOFMANN FOUNDATION

Founders: Oscar Janiger, M.D., Robert Zanger, M.A., President: Ron Brettin, 1278 Glenneyre St., No. 173, Laguna Beach, CA 92651 Tel 310/ 281.8110 Fax 714/497.0463.

THE HOFMANN FOUNDATION'S GOAL is to gather records of psychedelic research to advance the understanding and responsible application of psychedelics in investigating individual and collective consciousness.

A HOFMANN-MAPS-HEFFTER JOINT PROJECT

With the Heffter Research Institute and the Albert Hofmann Foundation, MAPS sponsors the WWW Psychedelic Research Bibliography, a no-charge, comprehensive, interactive bibliography on psychedelics and psychedelic research. Access it through graphical WWW browsers like Mosaic, Netscape and the browsers of America Online (AOL) and Netcom, and from these Web sites:

MAPS **HTTP://WWW.MAPS.ORG**
Heffter Research Institute **HTTP://WWW.HEFFTER.ORG**

Most researchers can access the National Library of Medicine's Medline database, but it only covers articles from 1966 to the present, and many domestic and foreign publications before 1966 aren't referenced electronically. The bibliography has 6,000 references to books and journal articles and is updated as resources like abstracts, graphics and full-text articles become available. It will be useful to researchers, students, libraries, federal officials and the psychedelically curious. The bibliography features full text and abstracts of articles no longer copyrighted or those the database has permission to reprint. Drugs listed in the archive include LSD, DMT, DPT, psilocybin, psilocin, ibogaine, harmaline, MDMA, MDE, MDA, mescaline and ketamine. The Psychedelic Research Bibliography includes:

MEDLINE

1966–1985	1986–1991	1992–1996

NAPRALERT

Biological activities of organisms	Hallucinogenic plants
Biological activities of chemicals	Euphoriant plants

References
Alkaloidal constituents per organism

Psychoactive plants

MDMA BIBLIOGRAPHY COMPILED BY ALEXANDER SHULGIN

Analytical methods

Animal toxicology

Biochemistry

Chemistry

Clinical studies

Human toxicology

In vitro studies

Legal history

Metabolism

Neurochemistry

Pharmacology

Reviews and social commentary

ASSORTED BIBLIOGRAPHIES

Ibogaine

Psychedelics and the dying

Aminorex

Ethnopharmacology

Native American peyotism

Central American Indians

South American Indians

Psychedelics in Western culture

Medical marijuana research bibliography by David Pate

Papers by David Nichols, Ph.D.

Papers by Alexander Shulgin, Ph.D.

Papers by Rick Strassman, M.D.

 Rick Strassman on

THE (NEAR) FUTURE OF PSYCHEDELIC RESEARCH

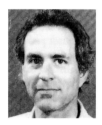

"The numbers of psychiatrists in the field of hallucinogen research is relatively small, and few apply for permission to study hallucinogens. Most older psychiatrists in academic and research psychiatry are pretty well established and wouldn't want to change fields, particularly to one that's controversial. In terms of the younger generation of psychiatrists, I think it's more a matter of ignorance than anything else. Younger psychiatrists don't know hallucinogens were in the mainstream of psychiatric research for 10 or 15 years after they were discovered, and that quite a few centers around the country were doing therapeutic and psychopharmacological research with psychedelics. So psychiatry ought to take some of the blame for [the 20- or 25-year gap] in human hallucinogen research, and psychiatrists in training should get more information about them.

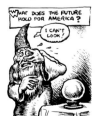

"[To summarize the resumption of human research with hallucinogens,] one can say that we're finishing up the first stage, [which] involved being able to establish a protocol for working with the government to get permission and funding to study these drugs in humans, to demonstrate that the drugs could be given safely to humans, and to begin some new psychopharmacology work. Now I think we're starting the second stage, which will involve studying the therapeutic applications of hallucinogens in people with psychiatric problems like alcoholism, substance abuse, terminal illness and post-traumatic stress syndrome (PTSD). All three conditions are hard to treat, have limited pharmacotherapy and showed promise in the first stage of psychedelic research."

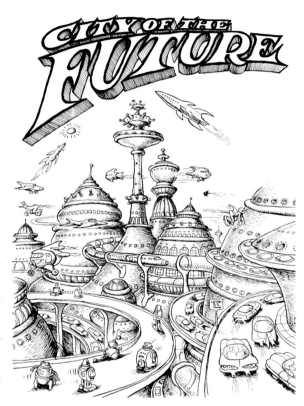

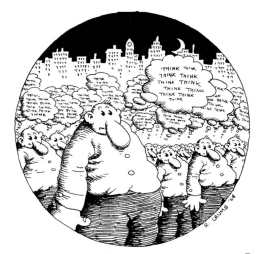

Chapter 12

THINK OR DIE:
THE REAL PROBLEM WITH HALLUCINOGENS

"I'm not afraid."—Luke Skywalker

"You *will* be."—Yoda

A CENTRAL PROBLEM with hallucinogens is that they aggravate the national multiple personality disorder whenever someone tries to do something—anything—about drugs. Legalize them, wipe them off the face of the earth, whatever. Alcohol, nicotine and caffeine are psychoactive drugs that create, depending on who you ask, billion-dollar megacorporations and lots of American jobs, hordes of helpless addicts who'd do anything to protect their source or platoons of teenaged puppet-zombies who exist to serve industry icons like Joe Camel, the Marlboro Man and all the young women who've come a long way. Baby.

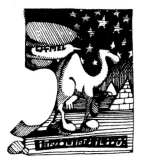

You won't find alcohol, nicotine or caffeine on any drug schedule (yet) either, but you will find marijuana under Schedule I, a category DEA reserves for drugs that have a high abuse potential, no currently accepted medical use in treatment in the U.S., and no accepted safety standards for use under medical supervision. Applied to the marijuana plant, these statements—to use an insult physicist Wolfgang Pauli (1900–1958) supposedly fired at one graduate student's groundless theory—aren't even *wrong*.

They actually sound a lot like the dialogue in *Reefer* Madness*,[144] a 1936 documelodra-ma-horror-fantasy, made with help from the FBI and shown in theaters as Truth:

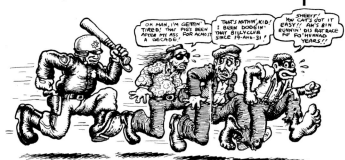

"Don't pass up a chance to see this pioneer effort in the government's anti-marijuana campaign," the video cover screams, **"made in 1936 in close collaboration with the F-B-I !"**

And drools, **"Reefer Madness shows how one puff of a marijuana cigarette can lead Clean-Cut Teenagers down the road to INSANITY & DEATH!"**

And howls, **"A moment of bliss. A lifetime of REGRET! Hunting a thrill, they inhaled A DRAG OF CONCENTRATED SIN!!!"****

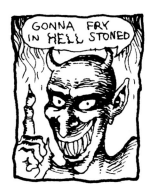

*Reefer is an old name that some people still use when discussing marijuana. It probably comes from the nautical term, reef. To reef a sail means to make it smaller by tucking in a part of the sail and tying it to or rolling it around a yard or pole attached to the mast. So the sail rolled around the yard looks like a rolled joint. A reefer was someone like a midshipman who reefed a lot of sails.

**Oh great. Marijuana has 61 cannabinoids including THC; 400 sugars, fats and acids; AND concentrated sin. Good luck isolating and synthesizing that. No wonder some people think DEA's blocking medical marijuana at the federal level.

So DEA and FDA officials think marijuana has no accepted medical use. Sure, except for 5,000 years in the Chinese pharmacopeia. And 100 or so years in the *U.S. Pharmacopeia* as a treatment for asthma, pain, seizures, sedation, muscle relaxation and anorexia. It was there until 1937, anyway, when public concern that one hit of marijuana would instantly turn smokers into heroin addicts led to the Marijuana Tax Act and the ban on recreational *and* medical marijuana use.

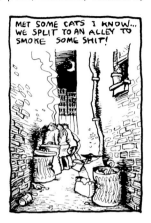

In the 1980s, some pharmaceutical company researchers got approval to test synthetic THC in animals and humans. In the lab researchers gave the mice *oral* doses of THC (actually smoking the joints singed their whiskers). Now THC's a Schedule II drug. That means it's available by prescription even though it's classified as having an approved medical use *and* a high potential for abuse. In 1985, synthetic THC got FDA approval as an antinausea agent for cancer patients. In December 1992, the FDA approved it to help fight weight loss (wasting) in AIDS patients. And some doctors supposedly prescribe synthetic THC to treat glaucoma, even though the FDA hasn't approved marketing the drug for that use. Lots of doctors and researchers say smoking marijuana can be more therapeutic than THC alone for patients with multiple sclerosis, AIDS, glaucoma, cancer and other diseases. And 35 states have passed legislation or resolutions that recognize marijuana's medical value.[145] But it's still a crime in the United States to smoke a joint.

So *there's* a problem—that hallucinogens and probably any drug, as Timothy Leary used to love explaining, people use for pleasure are psychotomimetic (psychosis-mimicking). In this case, that means they cause behavior that seems psychotic in people who *don't* use them, including many federal law enforcement and regulatory agency officials. But that's not the only problem.

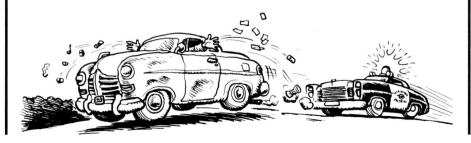

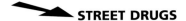

KID CHARLEMAGNE

While the music played, you worked by candlelight
Those San Francisco nights
You were the best in town
Just by chance you crossed a diamond with a pearl
You turned it on the world
That's when you turned the world around

Did you feel like Jesus
Did you realize
You were a champion in their eyes?

On the hill the stuff was laced with kerosene
But yours was kitchen clean
Everyone stopped to stare at the technicolor motorhome
Every A-frame had your number on the wall
You must have had it all
You'd go to LA on a dare
And you'd go it alone

Could you live forever
Could you see the day
Could you feel your whole world fall apart and fade away

Get along, get along Kid Charlemagne
Get along Kid Charlemagne

Now your patrons have all left you in the red
Your low-rent friends are dead
Life can be very strange
All those Day-Glo freaks who used to paint their face
They've joined the human race
Some things will never change

Son you were mistaken
You are obsolete
Look at all the white men on the street

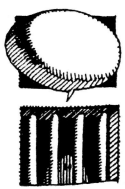

Clean this mess up else we'll all end up in jail
Those test tubes and the scale
Just get it all out of here
Is there gas in the car
Yes, there's gas in the car
I think the people down the hall know who you are

Careful what you carry
'Cause THE MAN is wise
You're still an outlaw in their eyes

from *The Royal Scam*, Steely Dan (Donald Fagen, Walter Becker), MCA Records Inc., Universal City, CA, 1976.

ANOTHER BIG PROBLEM with hallucinogens starts the first time some shaman buys psychedelic root scrapings from the wrong hunter-gatherer and goes *way* past his usual stop on the spirit-world train. Yeah. Street drugs. Just like reality— you never know what you're putting in your mouth or where it's been.

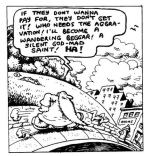

Back in the '60s, Haight-Ashbury was the United States' first in-your-face, open-air, one-stop shop for drugs—anything you could think of—and the first place (besides Sandoz in Basel) you could buy LSD like you'd buy brown rice or sod grass, in bulk. Lots of people made money there, but no one was a bigger cosmic success than the legendary (even then) Augustus Owsley Stanley III, featured esoterically in Walter Becker-Donald Fagen's "Kid Charlemagne."

LSD was still legal in 1964 when he and Berkeley chemistry major Melissa Cargill put their first product on the streets. Later, Owsley and Tim

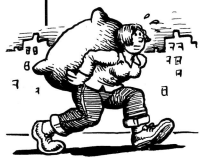

Scully, a Berkeley science dweeb with a geostationary IQ, set up an underground lab in Point Richmond, California, near San Francisco. Owsley was obsessed with making his product pure— definitely purer than Sandoz's yellowish crystalline LSD. It didn't take him long to find a way to refine the crystal so it looked blue-white under a fluorescent lamp. At first Owsley made LSD powder and measured it into gelatin caps. Later he produced it as a blue liquid so distributors could keep track of their sugar cubes.

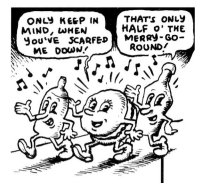

But it was hard to control the dose that way so Owsley bought a professional pill press and dyed the pills a different color every time he cranked out a shipment. Each tab had exactly 250 micrograms of LSD, even though each color had a different name—Yellow Sunshine, Purple Haze, Blue Cheer—and each was said to produce a different kind of trip.* Other acid was available but everyone knew Owsley's was the best and cleanest, and he held the price at $2 a hit. There was money in it but that wasn't his trip. He didn't sell drugs, he raised consciousness. He *believed* in LSD.[146]

➤ OWSLEY ON CLANDESTINE CHEMISTRY[147]

"I do not consider psychedelics a drug. You don't take it as an escape. You don't take it to cure something... In all the ethnobotanical matrices, in the cul-

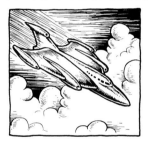

tures of Central and South America and... Africa, it's always used in a religious or a quasi-religious way... I found [taking LSD] kind of scary... like a crash course in how to become a jet pilot when you'd never seen a jet... They dropped you in there, took you up and said, *The controls are yours!* [maniacal laugh] Whoa! Barrel rolls! Immelmanns! Tailspins! Right into the ground sometimes. But psychically you recover from all this... if you're tough. I guess most of us were. [LSD] didn't come with a shaman who had 1,000 years or 10,000 years or 100,000 years of traditions and a ring of people holding your hand to show you the right way to go... I didn't know any more than anyone else, right? All I knew was that it was better to take a known substance in a known quantity than an unknown mixture of who-knows-what at god-knows-what quantity... I never told any-

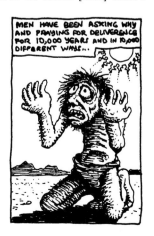

---

*Of course, each trip *was* different but that was always true of LSD, whose effects, like those of other hallucinogens, depend so heavily on set, setting and mood.

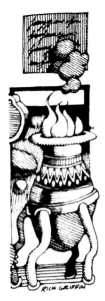

body to go out and take it... but I... wanted to take it... and I didn't want to poison myself. I didn't like Russian roulette with chemicals.[148]

"I put my hand on the reaction vessel during the procedures to put my energy in, to focus it so it could be the best it could be and then I would work very, very carefully to purify it to the point where I'd throw away 20 percent because to get the cleanest out, some of it couldn't be recovered... The total amount was so small that you would die if you knew how little I ever actually produced... probably more than that gets made every week now."[149]

The '60s produced a handful of spiritually advanced street chemists like Owsley, and a few smugglers and high-level drug dealers who were at least moderately motivated by idealism and radical politics. Even the Feds at DEA noticed: "It appears that the illicit production of dangerous drugs has become an intellectual and professional challenge to many individuals associated with [hallucinogen] misuse."[150]

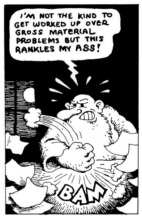

Changing times, new laws and life took their toll on the idealists, who were replaced by dealers out to make a profit. Chemically, LSD's not that complicated. If you do the reaction in a typical organic chemistry lab, it's considered routine—they say. But LSD's a little awkward to manufacture in secret. It calls for several hard-to-get 'watched' chemicals and a moderately sophisticated lab setup. Lab busts don't happen too often and consumption's been steady at tens of millions of hits a year since the late 1960s. Before you run out and set up a drive-thru LSD franchise, though, you should know that just buying

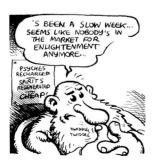

or trying to buy lab equipment or chemicals can be considered suspicious unless you're buying through a legitimate company or educational institution. Apparently cash, money orders and fake letterheads don't work anymore.

Nowadays the drug literature says people in the U.S. who manufacture controlled substances like LSD tend to be involved with organized, for-profit professional gangs.[151] They're not spreading enlightenment, they're exercising their right to make the best living they can in a free market economy. I guess that means no one puts their hands on the reaction vessels anymore.

A MEDICINAL CHEMIST ON STREET DRUGS

At the Medical College of Virginia in Richmond, medicinal chemist and psychopharmacologist Richard Glennon has studied psychedelics and their effects on the brain since the late 1960s. Like most hallucinogen researchers, he's into his work—all the monohydroxylated dimethyl heptyl homologs and nonselective 5-HT/dopamine agonists and structure-activity-related relationships between this and that ring-substituted phenylethylamine. But I wonder sometimes when I talk to scientists whether they ever look up from the rat lever box or lean back from the oscilloscope tracings and maybe rub their eyes and think about the people who use the drugs they study. The answer's yeah, they do.

"I feel sorry for them," Glennon said, "first of all that they're buying drugs off the street. No way in hell would I go and buy something from somebody on a street corner and shoot it up. I'm not even too fond of taking prescription drugs. I have two slides I use in a lot of my talks to high school kids or lay audiences or undergraduates. One is a schematic of drug development [that illustrates] what a drug has to go through before it appears on the market. From idea to design to development to testing and retesting and toxicity studies and pharmacology. There are all these boxes and you can follow arrows to all these other boxes.

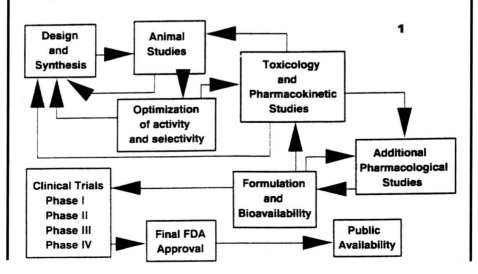

Synthesis	▶	Public Availability

2

SOURCE: DR. RICHARD GLENNON

The other slide shows one box—the idea—with an arrow to the street. You see something like that and realize that you could be the first human ever to take this drug. You don't know what you're buying on the street. There's no way to know. You have no idea what it's going to do. Do you really want to take that risk?

"In some cases the risks are real. MPTP is a byproduct of the synthesis of China White [synthetic heroin] that destroys dopaminergic neurons. Some people who took it got a Parkinson's-like syndrome and wento into catatonia. It's not psychoactive per se, it just destroys neurons. But who knows how many times this happens every day on the street, and the newspapers report it as so and so died of an overdose. How do you know what so and so died from? That's why I feel sorry for people who take street drugs.

"I don't advocate drug use. I don't advocate abstaining from drugs. I'm neutral on the issue. I like alcohol in moderation, I have no problem with it. At least you have some idea where it's coming from and I don't buy moonshine. But street drugs are a big problem and there should be more warnings about them. The drugs are bad enough, but you don't even know what you're getting when you buy stuff on the streets. That's certainly what I discussed with my kids when they were younger and I think they both turned out okay.

"What people do with their lives is their business," Glennon added, "but they should be as well-informed as they can possibly be and make educated choices."

◣ I KNOW WHAT YOU'RE THINKING...

How can you be well informed when nobody really has any idea about the long-term effects of hallucinogen use on the brain?

You can start with stuff they *do* know. The resources in this book alone would generate more drug information—good and bad—than anyone ever

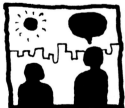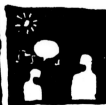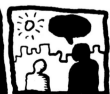

had time to read. There's literally no end to the drug bibliographies, archives, frequently asked questions (FAQs), Web sites, servers, home pages, news groups, chat groups, links and databases freely accessible on the Internet. There are libraries, 24-hour toll-free drug hotlines, 12-step programs, rehabs, detox centers and foundations for all kinds of addictions and compulsions. And there are informal ways to assess your vulnerability to certain drugs. All kinds of people need information about drugs, not just the ones who crash and burn. Addiction isn't the only end product of drug use, and that's the *real* point. You could start by listening to researchers like psychiatrist and neuropharmacologist Rick Strassman, who's spent a career thinking about hallucinogens and how they work in *your* brain.

➤ HALLUCINOGENS AREN'T FOR EVERYONE

"If someone with really high or low natural concentrations of serotonin took LSD," Strassman said during a September 1996 telephone interview, "I don't think it would matter a lot. But it *could*, I suppose, depending on one's normal levels of serotonin in the brain. It could have something to do with people being more or less sensitive to [a hallucinogen]. In our studies we gave DMT to around 60 people; two had almost no response on the same high dose everyone else got. I thought it was because of some difference in serotonin levels or the affinity of their serotonin receptors for DMT. Or it may be because they have fairly high serotonin levels in their brains in the first place. Either one—the factors are related.

"The state of receptors in the brain depends on concentrations [of neurotransmitters] floating around, and concentrations [of neurotransmitters] floating around depend on the receptor structure and its affinity for DMT. So serotonin concentrations and the functionality of the receptors for serotonin are in a fairly dynamic relationship. If someone had a history of psychotic

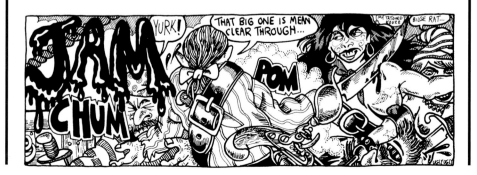

IS THIS YOU ???

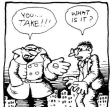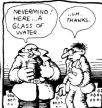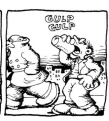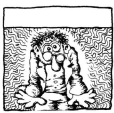

episodes [experiencing hallucinations or delusions is the hallmark of psychosis, and serotonin may have a role] independent of past drug use, I would flatly exclude that person from our studies.

"In people with histories of schizophrenic episodes, it's possible that exposure to psychedelics might precipitate a recurrence. If that person's serotonin system was unstable in the first place and you could disturb it even more with a psychedelic," Strassman added, "you might be asking for serious trouble. Some schizophrenics can become more floridly psychotic after exposure to a psychedelic. Some of the new antipsychotic medications like risperidone and clozaril have quite potent serotonin-blocking properties. It's a little more questionable in terms of a family history of psychosis. If a person was never psychotic themselves, one might be able to make a case for quite carefully administering a psychedelic in a particular research protocol. But it's still more prudent to avoid psychedelics in people with family histories of psychosis.

"Most schizophrenics start demonstrating symptoms in their late teens or early 20s. I would never give a 14-year-old a psychedelic, especially if they had schizophrenic parents. In our studies anyway, we need people to be at least 21 years old. I wanted to make certain there was no history of psychotic episodes in their lives, and I was also interested in their current level of social and vocational functioning, which starts becoming clear only after people leave home. All my volunteers were quite healthy, from psychiatric and physical points of view," he concluded. "I just didn't want to take any chances."

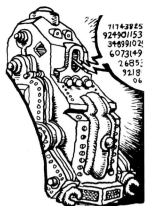

HERE ARE A COUPLE OF THINGS to think about if you take or are thinking about taking hallucinogens. Some people are more vulnerable than others to drugs, and some can be especially vulnerable to hallucinogens. I'm talking bad trips rather than addiction, because classic hallucinogens aren't linked with the drug reward system that's implicated in dependence on drugs like cocaine and speed.

I'm not a doctor. I'm not saying that if you do these things you can safely take LSD or anything else. This isn't a prescription, a recommendation, a suggestion, a hint or a clue. In fact, let's just say you can't safely put anything in your mouth, in a muscle or in a vein, under any circumstances. But if you do intend to use drugs, it can't hurt to know a couple of things.

🐌 People who tend to have bad trips are those who have family and personal histories of mental (neurochemical) instability. That's one reason it's *good* to know your immediate family's medical and mental health histories, at least through your grandparents and their brothers and sisters. This isn't always easy. Sometimes your information sources will lie through their teeth because they're in denial or because it's so uncool to have addicted, suicidal or mentally unstable relatives. Some might not even know they're passing along lies because no one in the extended family was ever allowed to mention crazy, drunk or psychotic relatives outside the immediate family.

🐌 Other people who tend to have bad trips are those who take any drug that's handy in any combination. These people should try very hard not to take handfuls of drugs all at once. If you do take drugs, take one at a time, take as low a dose as you can, as infrequently as you can. And—though this is almost impossible with street drugs—try to make sure the drug you think you're taking is the drug you're really taking, at the dose you expected. If you can't *not* take the drug, and you can't take any of the above precautions, try to use near

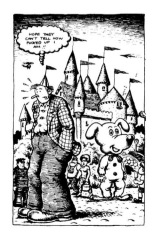

a major metropolitan hospital, trauma center or morgue.

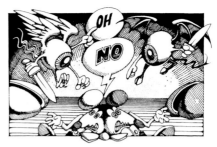

☺ Once you know or suspect your likely or potential physical and mental vulnerabilities, try to get a working knowledge of the brain—how it responds to different kinds of drugs and how you react to your brain's response to *any* drug—whether you make it yourself or get it over the counter at a drug store, from a doctor or your mother, from friends or drug dealers on the street.

☺ If you're vulnerable to mood swings, depression or other neurochemically based problems and you take antidepressants to control them, you'll want to be especially careful about taking other drugs at the same time. In Chapter 8, pharmacologist Katherine Bonson described the results of her study of people who mix antidepressants and hallucinogens. Those who took hallucinogens with serotonin reuptake blockers (SSRIs) or monoamine oxidase (MAO) inhibitors had a decreased or no response to hallucinogens. People who took tricyclic antidepressants or lithium had a much-increased response to hallucinogens and some had very bad adverse psychological effects. Lots of people who combined MDMA (ecstasy) and an MAO inhibitor had near-fatal responses because MDMA is a modified amphetamine and you should never mix stimulants and MAO inhibitors. But the bottom line is this: no one can predict what'll happen if you combine one drug with another.

➤ HAPPY TRAILS

The good news about hallucinogens is the bad news. LSD and other classic hallucinogens work in your brain because they look so much like natural neurotransmitters! And they're made right in the brain! No drug dealers, no contaminated batches, no busts! And they fit right into the same receptors! What's the problem?

It's mainly all that joint occupancy going on between hallucinogens and neurotransmitters at

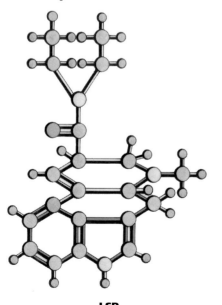

LSD

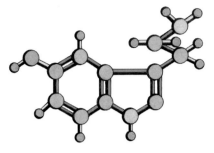

SEROTONIN (5-HT)

the receptor sites. Serotonin, dopamine and norepinephrine are neurotransmitters—major brain chemicals. Ancient systems, some of them, that may have existed even before sex, which originated a billion years ago, probably on a Saturday night, with blue-green algae and pond scum (but that's another story). The same systems that mediate your response to hallucinogens mediate your interaction with the universe. They make up your very own—

JUST ONE PER CUSTOMER—bio ultra critical graphical user interface (GUI, pronounced 'gooey'). The thing that integrates you and reality, that gives substance and meaning to everything you see and feel and touch and know.

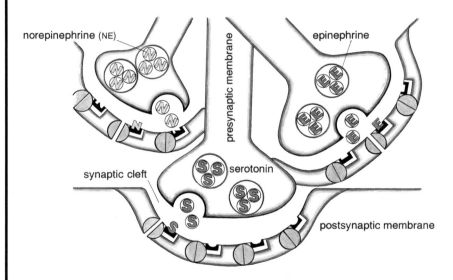

Dopamine may regulate body movement—walking, repetitive motions, feeding, drinking and probably is involved in the brain's reward system and addiction. The autonomic nervous system's sympathetic nerves may use norepinephrine to control emergency responses like accelerating the heart, dilating bronchi in the windpipe and raising blood pressure. Serotonin may help regulate sleep, memory, learning, body temperature, mood, behavior (including sex), cardiovascular function, the endocrine system (hormones) and pain perception. So, as the old Certs commercial used to say, it's 2... 2... 2

bummers in 1 if something goes horribly wrong—if the drug's contaminated or toxic; if someone sells you a dose that's more like 9 hits than 1; or if there's so much depression, psychosis and schizophrenia among your first-order relatives that locked wards make you feel all cozy and warm inside. Any of these could be some *bad* news if you use hallucinogens without knowing everything you can about them, and about yourself.

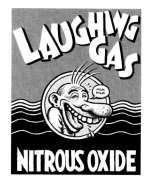

That's what's involved in deciding whether or not to use LSD, DMT, mescaline, psilocybin, MDMA. It's a serious decision and it's all yours. You *need* to know how hallucinogens and other drugs work in your brain. You'll have to work for it, though, because street drugs don't come with instruction diagrams, 24-hour toll-free hot lines, tech support or guarantees. And no one's going to make it easy for you. Especially people at school, at home, in Congress or at work who don't want you or anyone else using any drugs that they don't use and approve of.

You have to do it yourself and there's one requirement. Don't **JUST SAY NO** to drugs. Don't **JUST SAY YES**, either. Make up your own mind and do it the hard way: dig, investigate, examine, study, interview, debate, decide. You'll learn how to learn in the process, and it'll change your mind. You'll need it, too. Maybe thinking for themselves wasn't something Nancy Reagan's generation aspired to, but no one in the 21st century will have that luxury—nothing's getting any slower, easier, safer, cheaper or simpler.

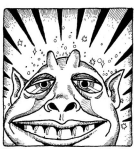

THE CHECKERED DEMON JUST SMILED.

◤ HELL FREEZES...

That's about when federal authorities, counselors, parents, teachers, doctors, professors, judges and cops will have credibility again with people who choose to use drugs. Andrew Weil, M.D., said it earlier in the book: "Since 1968 I have not met a single hallucinogen user who believes any reports of medical damage associated with drugs."[152]

Today, 30 years later, it's still tough to find a believer, mainly because nothing's changed. That's according to Joel Brown, Ph.D., MSW, author of "Drug Education and Democracy [In]action,"[153] a 1996 study of California's Drug, Alcohol and Tobacco Education (DATE) programs.

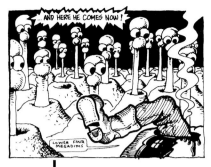

Random survey results from more than 5,000 adolescents showed that only 15 percent felt strongly and positively affected by drug education by the time they reached high school. To them, drug education is a small part of curricula with a huge negative effect on adult credibility, mainly because drug 'education' is really one message—substance use equals abuse. Outside school, though, students see others using drugs and having fun with no problems. Now they're in conflict, mistrustful of educators, and have no data for making their own substance use decisions. The students' disbelief is perpetuated.

But there is a way for educators, law enforcement officers, legislators and parents to end the cycle of mistrust. What could be so powerful? The other side of **JUST SAY NO**. The rest of the story. Words parents, educators and others are sure would send their students, their fellow citizens, their constituents, their kids swarming into the streets like starving dogs, looking for drugs.* It's nearly impossible for them to believe that...

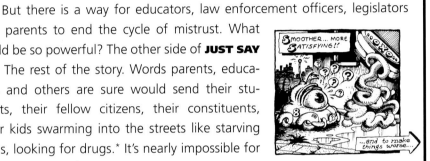

◎ All drugs aren't all bad for all people all the time.

◎ Not everyone who takes a drug—even a really powerful one like crack—gets addicted.

◎ Drugs aren't addictive all by themselves—they need people with the right neurochemistry to hook into and bleed dry. And everyone's brain chemistry is different for all kinds of reasons, including genetics, environment, diet and activity levels.

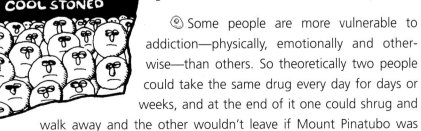

◎ Some people are more vulnerable to addiction—physically, emotionally and otherwise—than others. So theoretically two people could take the same drug every day for days or weeks, and at the end of it one could shrug and walk away and the other wouldn't leave if Mount Pinatubo was

*Classical hallucinogens like LSD and mescaline aren't addictive, but I mention it because so many people associate all drugs with addiction.

erupting behind him if he thought someone was on the way with more drugs.

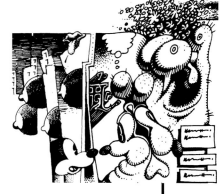

◉ Researchers are just *starting* to see how addiction and some kinds of drugs *might* work in the brain. And that means that today nobody—DEA, FDA, drug dealers, celebrities, rock stars, friends or people with Ph.D.s or M.D.s after their names or badges on their chests—knows exactly how or why drugs are good or bad in relation to your individual vulnerability.

◉ Some drugs are more toxic and risky than others.

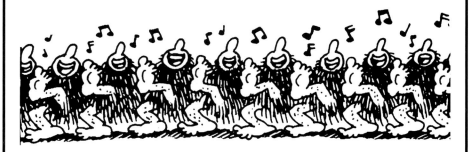

◉ Drugs *do* change people's minds but not always in bad ways.

◉ Some people have fun, socialize, relax, get closer to their spiritual beliefs, know themselves better and understand other people or start to see the world in a broader context, not just in terms of their own beliefs or country or planet. They use the drugs—not to excess—and stop when they've had enough or lose interest or whatever.

◉ Others were born without the little switch that tells them when something is enough. Some of these people could get 'addicted' to styrofoam if they were exposed to it under the right circumstances, and spend whatever's left of their lives trying to get more.

◉ Everyone else is somewhere between, and no quiz or blood test can predict who's who. That crap shoot called street drugs can probably tell you—if it doesn't kill you first. But take a close look at your family before you roll the dice.

TO EDUCATORS, LAW enforcement officers, legislators and parents, this is the terrifying, evil-twin, ax-murdering underside of JUST SAY NO: **not everyone who takes a drug ends up face down on the pavement.**

For them, nothing less than total abstinence from drugs is acceptable because they either don't trust people of *any* age to make their own decisions or they think all drugs are equally dangerous and addicting to anyone who gets too close. Either way, it's *ignore*-ance (ignorance), as philosopher Alan Watts[154] used to say, of drugs and the brain and the realities of both.

From my side of the bunker, spreading misinformation about LSD and the other hallucinogens is just as damaging as the Thalidomide-chromosome break rumors that survive today. The worst consequence of spreading misinformation is that it steals time and energy from the true job—making sure qualified researchers have access and permission to investigate the real problems associated with hallucinogens, and getting that information to as many people as possible.

That's what happened with hallucinogens and chromosome damage and flashbacks, and that's why I wrote *Trips*. Not to promote drug use or chemistry careers or to trash the Feds. But to describe in plain language, for anyone who's interested, what researchers are learning about psychedelics and the brain.

Some people won't get it because it's based on something they don't associate with drug information—the TRUTH.

Everyone else will need it where they're going—past the last exit before the toll plaza, under a new kind of warning sign (THINK OR DIE), heading into that 21st century.

And hey—whatever you decide about hallucinogens and other drugs, be *careful* out there.

"One way in which an increased knowledge of the... physical and biological world can be of value to the individual citizen is through conferring on him an increased equanimity—an increased confidence in natural law and order. The well-being of an individual may be greatly impaired by his fear of the unknown, which may far exceed the fear that he would have of a known danger, which he might prepare to meet in a rational way."—Linus Pauling (1901–1994), 1954 Nobel Prize/ chemistry; 1962 Nobel Peace Prize[155]

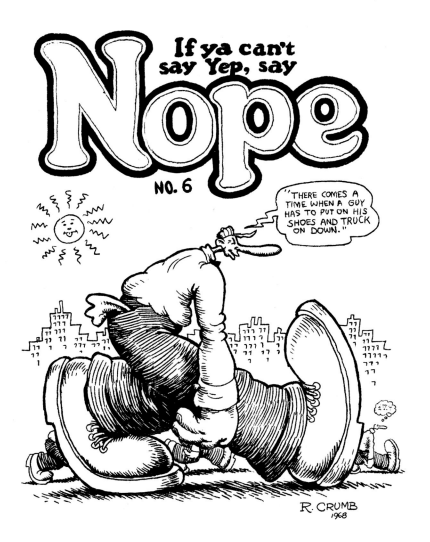

Other Stuff

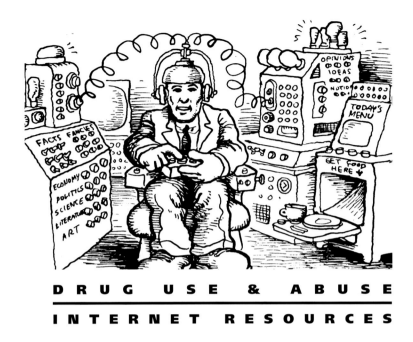

D R U G   U S E   &   A B U S E

I N T E R N E T   R E S O U R C E S

EVEN AS I POUND THIS OUT on the keyboard, some of the Web sites listed here are going off-line, moving or evolving into something else, somewhere else. Anyone familiar with the Internet already knows this, but please excuse any outdated information you find in this list of URLs (uniform resource locators). Here's more stuff about the Internet you probably already know:

DON'T BELIEVE EVERYTHING you read at any site (Duhhh...). In fact, here's a disclaimer from one Web site that's pretty standard on the net. Like they say, you use the Internet and everything on it at your own risk. Caveat emptor, you all.

DISCLAIMER Neither the server maintainers nor any contributors can be held liable in any way for any information or data made available or omitted from information distributed through this server. All the material may or may not have been checked for accuracy or completeness. All material is supplied "AS IS" without warranty of quality or

IF YOU WANT THE BEST, latest information on hallucinogens, try to use the best, most credible sources you can find. Figuring out how to tell the credible from the suspect sites takes knowledge, practice and sometimes the Psychic Hotline. In the meantime, if you want good basic information and research news about psychedelics, the brain and related stuff, I marked my favorites (★★) and the sites that have been especially useful in researching drugs (★★★). Others are probably just as good or better, but I haven't used them myself so I can't recommend them (★).

OTHER GOOD BETS ARE SITES sponsored by universities, science organizations and professional associations. Lots of Web sites are dedicated to drug dependence and addiction problems; you won't be surprised that these have sort of a *drug-use-is-abuse* slant, will you? And you'll find hundreds of other related resources—some are great, some blow. Just try to balance the Web sites of agencies like DEA, NIDA and the Partnership for a Drug-Free America against Web sites sponsored by guys with names like Blotterhead. Here's an intentionally noncomprehensive list of both.

★ **ADDICTION RESEARCH FOUNDATION**
http://www.arf.org/
The Addiction Research Foundation (ARF) is an agency of the Ontario Ministry of Health, established in 1949 to conduct research into alcohol, tobacco and other drug problems. It operates a central research and treatment facility in Toronto, 12 community program offices in centers across the province, and is a collaborating center of the World Health Organization.

★ **GUIDE TO ADDICTIONS INFORMATION ON THE INTERNET AND OTHER PUBLIC INFORMATION SITES**
http://www.arf.org:80/isd/links/mainpage.html
This list comes from the Addiction Research Foundation.

★ **THE ADDICTION TECHNOLOGY TRANSFER CENTER OF NEW ENGLAND**
http://center.butler.brown.edu/ATC-NE/
Formerly the Addiction Training Center of New England.

★ **CENTER FOR ALCOHOL AND ADDICTION STUDIES**
http://center.butler.brown.edu/index.html
Established at Brown University in 1982 to identify, prevent and treat alcohol and other drug use problems through research, publications, education and training.

★ ASSOCIATION FOR MEDICAL EDUCATION AND RESEARCH IN SUBSTANCE ABUSE
http://center.butler.brown.edu/AMERSA/

AMERSA (est. 1976) is an association of 400 health care professionals in the field of substance abuse whose goals are to 1) help make substance abuse education a required part of training for all health care professionals; 2) support research that has a multidisciplinary, multicultural approach to prevention, intervention and treatment; 3) distribute substance abuse information that emphasizes technology transfer, medical education and research through conferences and journals; and 4) support faculty development programs and help mentor health professionals who want to be teachers, clinicians and researchers in the field.

★ AMERICAN ACADEMY OF ADDICTION PSYCHIATRY
http://members.aol.com/addicpsych

Promotes excellence in clinical practice, makes quality treatment accessible to patients, and helps the public influence federal and state policies that involve addictive illness.

★ THE AMERICAN PSYCHIATRIC ASSOCIATION
http://www.psych.org

A national medical specialty society whose 40,500 physician members diagnose and treat mental and emotional illnesses and substance use disorders.

★ AMERICAN PSYCHOLOGICAL ASSOCIATION-DIV. 28
http://www.apa.org:80/divisions/div28/index.html

The home page of the APA division of psychopharmacology and substance abuse. Psychopharmacology combines psychology and pharmacology methods to study the effects of drugs on behavior. Research areas: behavioral pharmacology of psychoactive drugs, behavioral and pharmacological treatments of drug and substance abuse, clinical psychopharmacology, neurobehavioral toxicology, neurochemical mechanisms in substance abuse and related psychiatric disorders, the epidemiology of substance abuse.

★ AMERICAN SOCIETY FOR ADDICTION MEDICINE
http://www.asam.org

A medical specialty society dedicated to educating physicians and improving treatment for people with alcoholism and other addictions. Its goals are to improve access to care and increase its quality and effectiveness for patients and their families. The *Journal of Addictive Diseases* is published quarterly and is free to ASAM members.

★ CANADIAN CENTRE ON SUBSTANCE ABUSE
http://www.ccsa.ca/

CCSA is a nonprofit organization that works to minimize the harm associated with using alcohol, tobacco and other drugs. It offers, with McMaster University, distance education on the Internet—"Introduction to Substance Use and Abuse" is one Internet course offered.

★★ CENTER FOR ADDICTION & ALTERNATIVE MEDICINE RESEARCH
http://www.wInternet.com/~caamr/

The Center for Addiction and Alternative Medicine Research (CAAMR) is one of 10 research centers funded by the Office of Alternative Medicine (OAM) at the National Institutes of Health to promote promising treatments to consumers and doctors, and encourage communication among professionals involved in complementary and alternative medicine and substance abuse treatment. Complementary and alternative medicine includes mind-body control therapies, traditional and ethnomedicine, bioelectromagnetic therapies, diet and nutrition modification, body work and massage, and pharmacological, biological and energy therapies.

★ CENTER FOR DRUG RESEARCH
http://www.frw.uva.nl/acd/isg/drugs

The Center for Drugs Research (CEDRO—est. 1996) is a department of the School of Environmental Sciences at the University of Amsterdam. Its goal is to determine aspects of the drug problem from a socioscientific angle.

★ CENTER FOR EDUCATION AND DRUG ABUSE RESEARCH
http://www.pitt.edu/~mmv/cedar.html

The Center for Education and Drug Abuse Research (CEDAR) is funded by the National Institute on Drug Abuse (NIDA) to understand developmental factors that lead some people to normal life, some to drug abuse, and some to psychiatric problems. CEDAR is a consortium between the University of Pittsburgh and St. Francis Medical Center.

★ CENTER FOR SUBSTANCE ABUSE RESEARCH (CESAR)
http://www.csos.umd.edu/cesar/cesar.html

CESAR at the University of Maryland-College Park is a research center in the College of Behavioral and Social Sciences. The center collects, analyzes and distributes information on substance abuse; studies policies on preventing, treating and controlling substance abuse; and evaluates prevention and treatment programs. The CESAR Web site has weekly faxes on substance-abuse topics, biweekly faxes that evaluate drug treatment programs funded by the federal Center for Substance Abuse Treatment (CSAT), an electronic bulletin board that's (they say) one of the largest on-line sources of substance abuse information, and research reports and a substance abuse information clearinghouse.

★ CDC'S TOBACCO INFORMATION & PREVENTION SOURCEPAGE
http://www.cdc.gov/tobacco/

The sourcepage is maintained by the Office of Smoking and Health (OSH), a division in the Centers for Disease Control (CDC) and Prevention's National Center For Chronic Disease Prevention and Health Promotion.

★ CHANGE ASSESSMENT RESEARCH PROJECT
http://firenza.uh.edu/Departments. htmld/Psychology.htmld

Researchers at the Change Assessment Research Project have studied how people change since 1985. The project has two sites—Dr. Joseph Carbonari directs the program at the University of Houston in Texas; Dr. Carlo DiClemente directs the program at the University of Maryland-Baltimore County. The research is based on the Transtheoretical Stages of Change developed by DiClemente and researcher J.O. Prochaska. The transtheoretical model offers a framework for studying voluntary self- and therapy-assisted change. It describes underlying processes common to behavior change of all kinds but is most often used to assess change in behavior like smoking, alcohol abuse, condom use, exercise, diet and weight control.

THE TRANSTHEORETICAL MODEL

STAGES OF CHANGE: Precontemplation, contemplation, preparation, action, maintenance, termination.

PROCESSES OF CHANGE: Experiential processes, behavioral processes, consciousness raising, self-liberation, self-reevaluation, counterconditioning, dramatic relief, stimulus control, environmental, reevaluation, reinforcement, management, social liberation, helping relationships.

LEVELS OF CHANGE: Symptom or situational problems, maladaptive cognitions, current interpersonal conflicts or problems, family and system conflicts or problems, intrapersonal conflicts or problems.

★★ COUNCIL ON SPIRITUAL PRACTICES
http://www.csp.org/

The Council on Spiritual Practices (CSP) promotes drug reform from a spiritual perspective. It's dedicated to making direct experience of the sacred more accessible to more people. They say they do this by working peacefully and lawfully to identify and develop safe approaches to primary religious experience, and resolving social and legal obstacles to using certain drugs as religious sacraments.

★★ DENNIS MILLER HOME PAGE
http://www.hbo.com/dml

Website of the 1996 Emmy Award-winning *DENNIS MILLER LIVE* for... outstanding variety, music or comedy series and outstanding writing in a variety or music program. The king of sarcasm has hit the 'net.

★ DRUG DEPENDENCE RESEARCH CENTER, UNIVERSITY OF CALIFORNIA-SAN FRANCISCO
http://itsa.ucsf.edu/~ddrc

The Drug Dependence Research Center at the Langley Porter Psychiatric Institute, University of California-San Francisco focuses on the pharmacology, physiology and psychology of commonly abused drugs. The Web site has papers and posters, moments in psychopharmacological history, and information on San Francisco bay area drug treatment.

★★★ DRUG ENFORCEMENT ADMINISTRATION (DEA)
http://www.usdoj.gov/dea/deahome.htm

DEA is the lead federal agency for enforcing narcotics and controlled-substance laws and regulations. It maintains liaison with the United Nations, INTERPOL and other organizations on international narcotics control matters, and has offices across the U.S. and in 50 other countries.

★ LSD IN THE UNITED STATES. An excellent document from the DEA.
http://www.usdoj.gov/dea/pubs/lsd/toc.htm

★ FUTURE SYNTHETIC DRUGS OF ABUSE BY DONALD COOPER (DEA)
http://www.hyperreal.com/drugs/misc/future.html

In October 1987 the government amended the Controlled Substance

Act (CSA) to halt the development of designer drugs that looked and acted like controlled drugs but weren't chemically different enough to fall under the drug laws. DEA officials figure that kind of thing will keep happening, so they published this paper on drugs that might become designer drugs in the future. Cool.

★ SPEAKING OUT AGAINST DRUG LEGALIZATION
http://www.usdoj.gov/dea/pubs/legaliz/contents.htm

A guide developed by DEA.

★ DRUG REFORM COORDINATION NETWORK (DRCNET)
http://drcnet.org

DRCNet was founded in response to national drug policy. Their position is that the evidence on drug policy overwhelmingly favors decriminalization and reform is needed immediately. On this page they tell why the Drug War will end and offer supporting evidence. DRCNet hosts (they say) the world's largest on-line drug policy library.

★ DRCN LIBRARY
http://www.druglibrary.org

World's largest on-line drug policy library.

★ DRUG STRATEGIES
http://www.drugstrategies.org/

Drug Strategies is a nonprofit research institute that promotes better approaches to U.S. drug problems by supporting private and public initiatives that reduce the demand for drugs through prevention, education, treatment, law enforcement and community coalitions. Lots of publications for sale.

★ DRUGTEXT USA
http://www.drugtext.org/

The board of the International Foundation for Drug Policy and Human Rights publishes DrugText as part of its mission to promote development and dissemination of knowledge, research, education, scholarship and international jurisprudence in drug policy and human rights. Its first project was translating the German constitutional court decision on cannabis into English.

★ ECSTASY.ORG
http://www.ecstasy.org

E is for Ecstasy by Nicholas Saunders, bibliography by Alexander Shulgin, published 1993 by Nicholas Saunders, 14 Neal's Yard, London, WC2H 9DP, UK. ISBN: 0950162884, © 1994 Nicholas Saunders and Alexander Shulgin, 320 pages. Complete book on-line with references and bibliography; other books by Nicholas Saunders available by mail order.

★★ FEDWORLD
http://www.fedworld.gov/

The National Technical Information Service (NTIS) introduced FedWorld in Nov. 1992 as a central on-line access point for government information.

★★★ FOOD & DRUG ADMINISTRATION (FDA)
http://www.fda.gov

FDA regulates more than $1 trillion worth of products that account for 25 cents of every consumer dollar spent every year—food, cosmetics, medicines, medical devices, radiation-emitting products like microwave ovens, and animal feed and drugs. It also monitors product labeling and enforces the Federal Food, Drug and Cosmetic Act and other public health laws. The excellent, useful Web site has information on all this stuff.

★★ GOVERNMENT LINKS
http://www.eff.org/govt.html

International, national, regional and local governmental and government-related servers on the Internet.

★★★ HEFFTER RESEARCH INSTITUTE (HRI)
http://www.heffter. org

HRI was formed in 1993 to conduct excellent basic and clinical scientific research with psychedelic substances and disseminate the knowledge gained to the medical and scientific communities. It's named after Dr. Arthur Heffter, a turn-of-the-century German research pharmacologist who discovered that mescaline is the main psychoactive component in peyote cactus. Research findings and funding information from some of the premier scientists in the field.

★★ *HIGH TIMES* MAGAZINE
http://www.high times.com

The *High Times* Web site offers information on hemp, marijuana and psychedelic drugs (like LSD and ecstasy); cannabis cultivation; pot humor, drug laws, high art, drug tests and legal highs; industrial uses of hemp including hemp paper, clothing, foods, oil and others; legalization of marijuana, recreational use of marijuana, medical uses for marijuana, and worldwide uses for hemp and marijuana; articles from *High Times* magazine, an index of back issues, photographs of cannabis plants and information from the National Organization for the Reform of Marijuana Laws; and links to other hemp, marijuana and drug-related Web sites. The information is for adults only. *High Times* doesn't promote or condone the use of marijuana, alcohol, tobacco or other drugs. They ask that anyone who visits the Web site be at least 21 years old.

★★★ ALBERT HOFMANN, LSD: MY PROBLEM CHILD
http://www.dct.ac.uk/www/books/problem-child.html

Albert Hofmann's own account of his discovery of LSD, his career as a research chemist for Sandoz Pharmaceutical Co. in Basel, Switzerland, and the birth of the Psychedelic Age. He says that LSD, psilocybin and the other hallucinogens constitute cracks in the edifice of materialistic rationality that would benefit from exploration and maybe widening.

★ HOW TO RAISE DRUG-FREE KIDS
http://www.drugfreekids.com

The text here comes from a parenting guide, *How to Raise Drug-free Kids*, written by Per Ola and Emily d'Aulaire and created with the Partnership for a Drug-Free America, the U.S. Department of Education and ABC Television's *March Against Drugs*.

★★★ HYPERREAL
http://www.hyperreal.org

Hyperreal (main page and drug archive) is a collaborative publishing effort by more than 100 volunteers to give a home to alternative culture, music and expression. Special features include electronic publications, audio/video streaming resources, offsite links, independent dance label business resources, DARE—the straight dope on the U.S. antidrug program, a massive archive of information for electronic music (discographies, record label info, reviews, samples, artists, labels, mailing lists, music machines like synthesizers), Hyperreal's rave resources menu, techno-oriented chat room, Hyperreal media watch, an indispensable resource for unrestricted information about recreational drugs of all types, the Hyperreal Drugs Archives, and a small but useful library of sound and video tools including the ever-popular Acidwarp and links to related resources.

★ DRUG LINKS AT HYPERREAL—ENCYCLOPEDIC
http://www.paranoia.com:80/drugs/links/links1.html

★ *INTERNATIONAL JOURNAL OF DRUG POLICY*
http://www.xs4all.nl/~mlap/ijdp.html

Research, information and in-depth policy analysis of the global drug debate—legal, social, medical and educational issues related to using psychoactive substances. It focuses on the effects of drug policy and practice on drug-using behavior and its consequences, like HIV/AIDS, crime, law enforcement and social welfare. It's the journal's policy to reflect a wide range of beliefs and opinions on drug-related matters.

★ INTERNET MENTAL HEALTH
http://www.mentalhealth.com/

Internet Mental Health is a free encyclopedia of mental health information designed by Canadian psychiatrist Dr. Phillip Long for anyone interested in mental health. The Web site has information on the 50 most common mental disorders, treatment information for therapists, research, recovery stories, on-line diagnostic programs. articles and information for therapists on 65 of the most common psychiatric medications. *Mental Health Magazine* has news from the Internet and articles from professional and national magazines, newsletters and newspapers.

★ INTERPSYCH
http://www.psych.med.umich.edu/web/intpsych/

InterPsych is a nonprofit voluntary organization established on the 'net to promote international scholarly collaboration on research and intervention efforts in psychopathology. It offers scholarly electronic and real-time conferences, and plans to publish an e-journal. InterPsych has 8,000 members worldwide—anthropologists, computer scientists, neuroscientists, pharmacologists, philosophers, psychiatrists, psychologists and sociologists.

★ ISLAND GROUP
http://www.island.org

The Island Foundation is a nonprofit organization dedicated to creating a psychedelic culture and inspired by Aldous Huxley's novel, *Island*, about a utopian culture called Pala. It was founded in 1990 by Bruce Eisner and supported by memberships and contributions and sales from the Island Marketplace. The Island Foundation publishes *Island Views* newsletter, *Psychedelic Island Views* magazine, meets in e-groups to explore ideas they consider useful.

★★★ JOURNAL OF PSYCHOACTIVE DRUGS
http://mind.net/cns/jpd.htm

The *Journal of Psychoactive Drugs* was established in 1967 by David Smith, M.D., founder and medical director of the Haight-Ashbury Free Clinics. The journal is a quarterly periodical of multidisciplinary information on the use and abuse of psychoactive drugs. Topics have included the disease concept of addiction, drug use and criminality, drug use and the elderly, drug use and sexual behavior, ethnographic drug research, the history of cocaine smoking, therapeutic communities, hallucinogens, stimulants, depressants, smokable drugs, drug dependence and the family, women and substance abuse, professional treatment and the 12-step process.

★★ THE OFFICIAL DENIS LEARY WEB SITE
http://www.celebsites.com/DenisLeary/

Denis Leary's screamingly funny Web site, featuring the *Denis Leary 1997 Lock & Load Tour!*

★ TIMOTHY LEARY (1920-1997) HOME PAGE
http://www.leary.com

"Hello and welcome to my home! If you're a first time visitor, allow me take you on a guided tour." The guy talking is a digital version of the late Dr. Timothy Leary—controversial, influential psychologist, spiritual leader of the countercultural 1960s and 1970s, a promising young clinical researcher who helped develop the theory of transactional analysis and changed forever the doctor-patient relationship in modern psychology, conductor of a provocative series of psychedelic experiments at Harvard, fired from Harvard with Richard Alpert shortly after, prisoner for marijuana possession with a stiffer sentence than someone in for Murder-1, instigator of mischief during the era of cultural and psychosocial upheaval, phrasemaker, questioner of authority, explorer of alternative realities, creator of psychotherapeutic computer software (Mind Mirror), victim of fatal prostate cancer, celebrator of his own death, explorer of the consciousness of dying—with daring and humor. God[s] keep his soul.

★ HOW TO OPERATE YOUR BRAIN, TIMOTHY LEARY
http://www.leary.com/home/TVRoom/HowBrain.html

Information is power. Think for yourself. CAUTION: proper use of the brain is not endorsed by federal governments or huge corporations that profit from a brainwashed, enslaved population. Mild discomfort may occur as confusing independent thought challenges popular views of the world.

Using a mix of right-brain visual communication and left brain narration, Timothy Leary leads an intensely psychedelic, techno-hyperstimulated tour on how to guide yourself through all realms of perceptual consciousness—topics like chaos, creating your own realities, thinking for yourself, questioning authority, and the emerging techno–logical Global Village. This video accompanied his '93-'95 personal appearances. It seeks to create a state that overwhelms and intrigues the rational mind. Order on-line at this site.

★★★LINDESMITH CENTER
http://www.soros.org

The Lindesmith Center is a Manhattan-based policy research institute founded in 1994 that focuses on broadening the debate on drug policy and related issues. Center director is Ethan Nadelmann J.D., Ph.D., author of *Cops Across Borders: The Internationalization of U.S. Criminal Law Enforcement* (Penn State Press 1993). The Web site features full-text articles from the academic and popular press on drug policy from economic, criminal justice and public health perspectives. It has a seminar series, library and information center, and a grants program in central and eastern Europe. Its members take on special projects on topics like methadone policy reform and alternatives to drug testing in the workplace. The center's guiding principle is harm reduction, an alternative approach to drug policy and treatment that seeks to minimize adverse effects of drug use *and* prohibition. In 1996 the Center opened a San Francisco office directed by Marsha Rosenbaum Ph.D., a veteran National Institute on Drug Abuse grantee and author of *Women on Heroin* and other writings on drug use, drug abuse, drug education, women's issues and drug treatment. Contact Lindesmith[east] at 212/887/0695 or http://www.linde smith.org; Lindesmith[west] at 415/921/4987 or marsharose@aol.com.

★★★LYCAEUM
http://www.lycaeum.org/
Quote seen at the Web site:
"Be All That You Can Be!"—The U.S. Army

This awesome Web site has (they say [and I believe it]) the largest psychedelic drug library in the world, featuring Magic Mushrooms, marijuana, LSD, extraction manual, trip reports; more than 100 megabytes of graphics—psychedelic celebrities, visionary plants, visionary chemicals and psychedelic art; 22 free on-line psychedelic books, book reviews, company resources and an on-line entheogenic bookstore; more than 1,000 links to other drug sites around the world, FAQs, drug information, organizations; mind-melting computer software for your PC or Macintosh; on-line forums; drug war info, including an educational page about the government's failing policies; contests, fund raisers, FAQs, surveys and more; some excellent hosted WWW home pages on politics, drug information, products and supplies; and member account-management services.

★★★ THE MID-ATLANTIC ASSOCIATION OF FORENSIC SCIENTISTS (MAAFS)
http://www.gwu.edu/~fors/maafs/druglink.htm
Fascinating Web site. MAAFS forensic links—narcotics, universities, forensic chemistry, forensic labs, forensic conferences and meetings, forensic mailing lists, general forensic links, more general forensic links, related literature, forensic specialty sites, forensic anthropology, forensics and computers misc., forensic medicine, forensic imaging, question documents, new forensic links, drug links, forensic societies, national and international government forensic links, firearms, DNA.

★★★ MULTIDISCIPLINARY ASSOCIATION FOR PSYCHEDELIC STUDIES (MAPS)
http://www.maps.org/
Sponsors research the therapeutic applications of psychedelics and marijuana. The Multidisciplinary Association for Psychedelic Studies (MAPS) is a 501 (c) (3) corporation chartered in 1986 as a membership-based research and educational organization. Now with 1400 members, MAPS

focuses on developing beneficial, socially sanctioned uses of psychedelic drugs and marijuana—psychotherapeutic research and treatment, addiction treatment, pain relief, spiritual exploration, shamanic healing, psychic research, brain physiology research and related scientific inquiries. MAPS helps researchers design, get government approval for, fund, conduct and report on psychedelic research in human volunteers. It publishes a quarterly publication for members, government policymakers and academic experts; it funds FDA-approved human research with MDMA and works to initiate FDA-approved marijuana research. Access to past newsletters allows visitors to review the history and status of research on MDMA, psilocybin, DMT, ibogaine, ayahuasca, marijuana, LSD, ketamine and other drugs. The WWW Psychedelic Bibliography is a searchable electronic bibliography of scientific papers related to psychedelic drugs. It's funded by MAPS, the Heffter Research Institute and the Albert Hofmann Foundation.

★★★ MEDICAL SCIENCES BULLETIN (MSB)
http://pharminfo.com/pubs/msb/msbmnu.html

Medical Sciences Bulletin (MSB) is a source of high-quality information on drug therapies, related pharmacology and advances in the fast-moving field of clinical pharmacology. It's published bimonthly by Pharmaceutical Information Associates Ltd., Levittown PA as part of PharmInfoNet. Each MSB issue covers a specific therapeutic category and includes review articles on drugs as soon as they're approved or recommended for public use. Hundreds of archived articles from past issues form a searchable library of pharmaceutical information that's fairly accessible to a general audience. Drug categories are anti-infective drug reviews; anti-inflammatory, antiallergic and immunologic drug reviews; cardiovascular drug reviews; endocrine and metabolic drug reviews; gastrointestinal drug reviews; oncology drug reviews; ophthalmologic drug reviews; psychopharmacologic and neurologic (CNS) drug reviews; respiratory drug reviews; and miscellaneous drug reviews.

★ DUAL DIAGNOSIS WEB SITE
http://www.erols.com/ksciacca/

Someone with a dual diagnosis has co-occurring mental illness, drug addiction and alcoholism in various combinations. This site offers information and resources for doctors, consumers and family members who need help or education on the topic. The ultimate goal is to improve treatment systems that have evolved to address one problem at a time. The Web site has a glossary; clinical profiles; training opportunities and education and training events; and dual diagnosis literature, articles, chapters and abstracts.

★ HEALTHGUIDE: MENTAL HEALTH
http://www.healthguide.com/MHealth/

T. Bradley Tanner, M.D., is a clinical assistant professor of psychiatry in the Department of Psychiatry at the University of Pittsburgh School of Medicine. He's also president and chief executive of Clinical Tools Inc., a multimedia software firm that specializes in health education and offers health information and materials to the public through the Internet, and on CD-ROM software and videotape.

★ THE NATIONAL CENTER ON ADDICTION AND SUBSTANCE ABUSE AT COLUMBIA UNIVERSITY (CASA)
http://www.casacolumbia.org/

A resource for research on addiction and substance abuse. It provides access to information, research and commentary on tobacco, alcohol and drug abuse issues including prevention, treatment and cost data.

★★★ NATIONAL INSTITUTE ON DRUG ABUSE (NIDA)
http://www.nida.nih.gov/

The NIDA Web site is a great resource for information on the latest research on drugs and how they work in the brain, despite its inevitable all-drugs-are-bad-for-all-people perspective. NIDA says its mission is to bring the power of science to bear on drug abuse and addiction by supporting and conducting research across a range of disciplines, and by making sure those research results are quickly distributed to those involved in drug-abuse and addiction prevention, treatment, and policy.

★ INFORMATION ON DRUGS OF ABUSE
http://www.nida.nih.gov/DrugAbuse.html
Good information on specific drugs.

★ NIDA CAPSULES
http://www.nida.nih.gov/NIDACapsules/NCIndex.html
NIDA Capsules are fact sheets that summarize topics for the press and public that range from drug-abuse statistics to public education campaigns.

★ NIDA NOTES
http://www.nida.nih.gov/NIDA_Notes/NNindex.html

NIDA Notes is a bimonthly publication that covers treatment and prevention research, epidemiology, neuroscience, behavioral research, health services research and AIDS. It reports on advances in the drug-abuse field, identifies resources, promotes information exchange and seeks to improve communications among clinicians, researchers, administrators and policymakers. The *NIDA Notes Research Report Series* simplifies the science of research and reports on findings of national interest.

★ MONOGRAPH 159: INDIVIDUAL DIFFERENCES IN THE BIOBEHAVIORAL ETIOLOGY OF DRUG ABUSE [PDF FORMAT]
http://www.nida.nih.gov/pdf/monographs/monograph159/download159.html

★ NATIONAL CLEARINGHOUSE FOR ALCOHOL & DRUG INFORMATION (NCADI)
http://www.health.org

NCADI is the information service of the Center for Substance Abuse Prevention of the Department of Health and Human Services. The largest resource for substance abuse prevention information.

★★★ NATIONAL INSTITUTE OF ALCOHOL ABUSE & ALCOHOLISM (NIAAA)
http://www.niaaa.nih.gov/

NIAAA supports and conducts biomedical and behavioral research on alcoholism and alcohol-related problems. The site has full-text e-versions of *Alcohol Alerts*, a quarterly research report on alcohol abuse and alcoholism. Scary facts about what alcohol really does to the body and brain!

★★★ THE SOCIETY FOR NEUROSCIENCE
http://www.sfn.org/

The Society for Neuroscience is one of the world's largest organizations of scientists and physicians dedicated to understanding the brain, spinal cord and peripheral nervous system. Neuroscientists investigate the molecular and cellular levels of the nervous system; brain systems like vision and hearing; and behavior produced by the brain. Medical specialties in neuriscience include neurology, neurosurgery, psychiatry and opthalmology.

The society has grown from 500 members in 1970 to more than 25,000 members today. The society advances understanding of the nervous system by linking multidisciplinary scientists and encouraging research in all aspects of neuroscience, promoting neuroscience education, making the public aware of new research results and implications; and exchanging information at annual meetings of more than 20,000 participants from the Americas, Europe and Asia. It's an arena for presenting new neuroscience research and the site of courses, workshops and symposia for members. *The Journal of Neuroscience*, published twice a month, has articles on a range of neuroscience research. Other publications include *Brain Facts,* a 52-page primer on the brain and nervous system; *Brain Concepts,* a series of brochures on neuroscience topics; *Brain Briefings,* a series of newsletters explaining how basic neuroscience discoveries lead to clinical applications; *Brain Waves,* a newsletter on neuroscience advances for congressional staffers, and more.

★★★ PARANOIA'S DRUG INFORMATION SERVER
http://www.paranoia.com/drugs

Paranoia's Drug Information Server is a collection of usenet posts, e-mail contributions and private research on drugs and drug use. It's run by volunteers and is a good place to look for hard-to-find information on drugs. It also has real accounts of drug use experiences, good and bad. Visitors can add their own stories, anonymously if they want to, and there are extensive bibliographies and links to sites that range from NORML to the DEA.

★★★ PARTNERSHIP FOR A DRUG-FREE AMERICA
http://www.drugfreeamerica.org/

The Partnership for a Drug-Free America is a nonprofit coalition of professionals from the communications industry who aim to reduce the demand for illegal drugs through advertisements. They're the ones who did "This is your brain on drugs... " They formed in 1986 with seed money from the American Association of Advertising Agencies. They have a staff of 30 and volunteers from the media, advertising agencies, production houses, talent guilds, and research and public relations firms who donate advertising, broadcast time and print space for antidrug public service messages. They call their Web site "the largest, most accurate database of drug information on the web."

★ PATHOLOGY OF DRUG ABUSE
http://www-medlib.med.utah.edu/WebPath/DRUG.html

Minitutorial of some of the health risks of smoking, drinking alcohol, and using cocaine (with images).

★★★ STANTON PEELE'S ADDICTION WEB SITE
http://peele.sas.nl/

This is the Web site of Stanton Peele, a guy with controversial views about addiction and recovery. He has good credentials (Ph.D., social psychology, University of Michigan 1973; B.A., political science, University of Pennsylvania 1967; New Jersey Psychology License #1368), has won several awards (1994 Alfred Lindesmith Award from the Drug Policy Foundation, Washington D.C.; 1989 Mark Keller Award from the Rutgers Center for Alcohol Studies, New Brunswick NJ; and others), and holds impressive current positions (consultant, International Center for Alcohol Policies, Washington D.C., 1996-present; editorial board, *Addiction Research,* 1994-present; forensic psychologist, criminal responsibility, psychiatric and chemical dependence treatment abuses, 1987-present; advisor, American Psychiatric Association, DSM-IV section on substance abuse, 1992-1993). The Web site has FAQs, articles, Peele's curriculum vitae, an on-line library, and the full text of many of his articles. Visitors can send addiction questions to ASK STANTON, and get Peele's take on the meaning of the latest addiction research.

★★★ PHARMACEUTICAL INFORMATION NETWORK
(PHARMINFONET)
http://pharminfo.com/

PharmInfoNet provides pharmacological information about prescription or over-the-counter drugs as a free service to people with legitimate questions about their medications. PharmInfoNet works with a panel of medically qualified consultants—some are volunteers, others are paid—to help answer questions from readers and moderate e-mail discussion groups. PharmInfoNet doesn't give medical advice.

★ PHARMACOLOGY GLOSSARY
http://med-amsa.bu.edu/Pharmacology/Programmed/
glossary.html

Department of Pharmacology and Experimental Therapeutics, Boston University School of Medicine. A glossary of terms and symbols used in pharmacology.

★★★ **PHENETHYLAMINES I HAVE KNOWN AND LOVED (PIHKAL)**
http://www.bong.com/drugs/pihkal
Phenethylamines I Have Known and Loved, Alexander and Ann Shulgin's epic index (HTML version) of phenethylamines like DMT and mescaline.

★ **QUALITY HEALTH INC.**
http://www.qhi.co.uk
Quality Health Inc. is a mail-order source for pharmaceuticals, smart drugs, antiaging remedies and life extension medications at (they say) some of the best prices available.

★ **REALITY CHECK**
http://www.health.org/reality/index.htm
Reality Check is a public education campaign to counter a resurgence in marijuana use among teenagers. It's run by the federal Center for Substance Abuse Prevention (CSAP).

★ **SHRINKTANK BBS WEB SITE**
http://www.shrinktank.com/
Psychology and mental health software.

★ **SUBSTANCE ABUSE & MENTAL HEALTH SERVICES ADMINISTRATION (SAMHSA)**
http://www.samhsa.gov/
SAMHSA's mission is to make sure substance abuse and mental health services are available to people who need them through three centers— Mental Health Services, Substance Abuse Prevention and Substance Abuse Treatment—and offices that target applied studies, managed care for mental health and substance abuse services, AIDS, women's services. Most SAMHSA work is done through federal grants and contracts to state and local agencies and private service providers. Learn more about funding opportunities at this site's electronic bulletin board.

★ THE NATIONAL MENTAL HEALTH SERVICES KNOWLEDGE EXCHANGE NETWORK (KEN)
http://www.mentalhealth.org

KEN is a national, one-stop source of information and resources on prevention, treatment and rehab services for people with mental disorders. The National Center for Mental Health Services developed KEN for those who use mental health services, their families, the public, policymakers, providers and the media. This site has a database of on-line resources, toll-free telephone services, an electronic bulletin board and a catalog of free publications that can be ordered on-line.

★ UCLA DRUG ABUSE RESEARCH CENTER (DARC)
http://www.mednet.ucla.edu/som/ddo/npi/DARC

DARC is a research organization that investigates psychosocial and epidemiological issues of drug use and evaluates drug dependence interventions. DARC findings help develop more effective strategies for dealing with drug-related problems through prevention, treatment and criminal justice approaches. It's affiliated with the UCLA Neuropsychiatric Institute, a leading facilities for patient care, education and research in mental health and neurology. The center also distributes information on drug abuse and trains future researchers and scientists in related fields.

★★ WEB OF ADDICTIONS
http://www.well.com/user/woa

The Web of Addictions was established to make sure there was accurate information about alcohol and other drug addictions on the Internet. The developers say: "We developed the Web of Addictions for several reasons. We are concerned about the pro-drug-use messages in some Web sites and in some use groups. We are concerned about the appalling extent of misinformation about abused drugs on the Internet, particularly on some usenet news groups. Finally, we wanted to provide a resource for teachers, students and others who needed factual information about abused drugs. We have received several awards. We are proud of the recognition we have received because it enhances the credibility of the information presented in these pages. We take addictions seriously. You won't find glib, hip treatment of this very serious topic here."

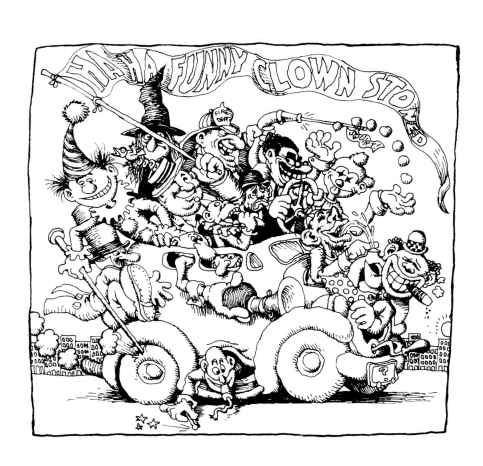

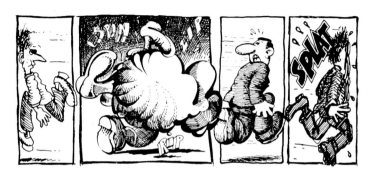

H A L L U C I N O G E N   P R O F I L E S

C L O C K I N G   Y O U R   G R O U N D   S P E E D

Ralph Metzner Ph.D., Altered States Graphic Profile;
Rick Strassman M.D., Hallucinogen Rating Scale

RALPH METZNER, Ph.D.
ALTERED STATES GRAPHIC PROFILE (ASGP)
© 1986. 2nd, revised edition

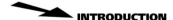 **INTRODUCTION**

The Altered States Graphic Profile (ASGP) is designed to assess and display in graphic form two major dimensions of altered states of consciousness—the level of arousal or wakefulness, and the pleasure-pain (hedonic) continuum. Individuals can, with a little advance preparation, give numerical estimates of these two aspects of awareness, regardless of the content of the experience and how the altered state is induced. This kind of measurement of subjective experience 1) can facilitate the individual's own observation, reflection and recollection of states of consciousness (experience shows that doing the rating helps ground people during new and confusing experiences) and 2)

permits comparative research on states of consciousness induced by different drugs or by hypnosis, meditation, sound, music, sensory deprivation, breathing, sex or movement. Research on how variables such as personality might affect altered states would also be possible with this ASGP.

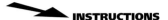 **INSTRUCTIONS**

Of the two separate graphs, the upper graph is for the arousal continuum, the lower for the hedonic (pleasure-pain) continuum. Every 15 minutes during the chosen time period, you assign a numerical value ranging from +3 to -3 to your subjective sense of these two dimensions. The ratings can be done at less frequent intervals, but both scales should always be scored. Actual clock-time hours can be entered in small boxes at the bottom of each graph. It is best to obtain at least an hour's worth of readings before the trigger event (drug ingestion) to serve as a baseline against the altered state values. The space between the two graphs can be used to show the time and nature of triggers and other external stimulus events that presumably affected the altered state. These might include 150 mg MDMA, one glass of wine, 3 lungfuls of marijuana, hypnotic induction, begin zazen sitting (Zen meditation), 20 minutes of symphonic music, chanting OM (meditation), watching a sunset, or relating to your partner. The experiencer can enter the ratings, or give them to a guide, sitter, therapist or friend who can enter them.

THE SCALES

The ratings called for are **numerical** estimates of your experience. The descriptive adjectives are rough indications whose meanings will vary from person to person. We assume that both these dimensions vary upward and downward from the presumed normal, usual or baseline midpoint of zero. The **arousal continuum** is a measure of wakefulness and attentiveness; it should be distinguished from the active-passive and tension-relaxation dimensions. Point -1 corresponds to EEG alpha waves and light hypnotic trance; point -2 to theta waves, twilight imagery with drowsy drifting and moderate trance; and -3 to deep trance or sleep or complete dissociation from the environment. On the **hedonic continuum**, the negative part of the scale includes negative emotional states such as anxiety, depression, anger or sickness. The intensity and pleasure or discomfort are being assessed, not specific emotions. You can indicate more specific information about the experience content in the space provided for listing trigger events.

Ralph Metzner, Ph.D.

ALTERED STATES GRAPHIC PROFILE (ASGP) FORM

©1986. 2nd revised edition

Name _____ Date _____

Sex _____ Date of Birth _____

I THE AROUSAL CONTINUUM

aroused/excited	+3			
stimulated	+2			
alert/attentive	+1			
awake & calm	0			
alpha/meditative	-1			
drifting/twilight	-2			
deep trance/sleep	-3			
indicate clock time		15	30	45

Indicate trigger and other external events

II THE HEDONIC CONTINUUM

ecstatic/heaven	+3			
elated/euphoric	+2			
pleasant	+1			
neutral	0			
unpleasant	-1			
painful/disturbing	-2			
agony/hell	-3			
indicate clock time		15	30	45

RICK STRASSMAN, M.D.

►HALLUCINOGEN RATING SCALE (HRS)

© 1990. Used with permission.

STRASSMAN AND HIS GROUP started developing the Hallucinogen Rating Scale (HRS)[156] by interviewing 19 experienced DMT users who'd also taken lots of other hallucinogens. Most were very educated and well-functioning. They smoked specific doses of free-base DMT (the usual for recreational use) and described the drug effects. The volunteers had a range of negative, positive and neutral experiences, but mostly they reported positive effects. This scale is different from other scales because it's not based on a particular theoretical framework; it's based on responses of people who have taken a lot of hallucinogens and can describe the full range of effects.

►HRS (VERSION 3.06)

Below is a list of statements referring to effects of the drug you received. For each statement, please mark the answer that corresponds to the most intensely you experienced that effect during the specified time period. For this questionnaire, answer for _____. Please mark only one answer for each item—the answer that seems best—even if none matches your experience exactly. Don't worry if your answers to some questions are opposite to others. If two opposite experiences occurred at some point during the time period, answer each one according to what you experienced.

Name_____ Date_____ Dose_____ Protocol_____ (Session_____)

1. Amount of time between drug administration and feeling an effect

N/A no effect	0-5 seconds	5-15 seconds	15-30 seconds	30-60 seconds	More than 1 minute

2. A rush

Not at all	Slightly	Moderately	Very much	Extremely

2a. Location of rush _____

3. Change in salivation

Not at all	Slightly	Moderately	Very much	Extremely

3a. Drier, wetter, or both (circle one)

4. Body feels different

Not at all	Slightly	Moderately	Very much	Extremely

4a. Please describe _____

  5. Change in sense of body weight

Not at all   **Slightly**   **Moderately**   **Very much**   **Extremely**

5a. Lighter, heavier, or both (circle one)

  6. Feel as if moving/flying through space

Not at all   **Slightly**   **Moderately**   **Very much**   **Extremely**

  7. Change in body temperature

Not at all   **Slightly**   **Moderately**   **Very much**   **Extremely**

7a. Warmer, colder, or both (circle one)

  8. Electric/tingling feeling

Not at all   **Slightly**   **Moderately**   **Very much**   **Extremely**

  9. Pressure or weight in chest or abdomen

Not at all   **Slightly**   **Moderately**   **Very much**   **Extremely**

9a. Physically loose, limber, or flexible

Not at all   **Slightly**   **Moderately**   **Very much**   **Extremely**

10. Shaky feelings inside

Not at all   **Slightly**   **Moderately**   **Very much**   **Extremely**

11. Feel body shake/tremble

Not at all   **Slightly**   **Moderately**   **Very much**   **Extremely**

12. Feel heart beating

Not at all   **Slightly**   **Moderately**   **Very much**   **Extremely**

13. Feel heart skipping beats or beating irregularly

Not at all   **Slightly**   **Moderately**   **Very much**   **Extremely**

14. Nausea

Not at all   **Slightly**   **Moderately**   **Very much**   **Extremely**

15. Physically comfortable

Not at all   **Slightly**   **Moderately**   **Very much**   **Extremely**

16. Physically restless

Not at all   **Slightly**   **Moderately**   **Very much**   **Extremely**

17. Flushed

Not at all   **Slightly**   **Moderately**   **Very much**   **Extremely**

18. Urge to urinate

Not at all   **Slightly**   **Moderately**   **Very much**   **Extremely**

19. Urge to move bowels

Not at all   **Slightly**   **Moderately**   **Very much**   **Extremely**

20. Sexual feelings

Not at all   **Slightly**   **Moderately**   **Very much**   **Extremely**

21. Feel removed, detached, separated from body

Not at all   **Slightly**   **Moderately**   **Very much**   **Extremely**

22. Change in skin sensitivity

Not at all   **Slightly**   **Moderately**   **Very much**   **Extremely**

22a. More sensitive, less sensitive, or both (circle one)

23. Sweating

Not at all   **Slightly**   **Moderately**   **Very much**   **Extremely**

24. Headache

Not at all   **Slightly**   **Moderately**   **Very much**   **Extremely**

25. Anxious

Not at all   **Slightly**   **Moderately**   **Very much**   **Extremely**

26. Frightened

Not at all   **Slightly**   **Moderately**   **Very much**   **Extremely**

27. Panic

Not at all   **Slightly**   **Moderately**   **Very much**   **Extremely**

27a. Self-accepting

Not at all   **Slightly**   **Moderately**   **Very much**   **Extremely**

27b. Forgiving yourself or others

Not at all   **Slightly**   **Moderately**   **Very much**   **Extremely**

28. At ease

Not at all   **Slightly**   **Moderately**   **Very much**   **Extremely**

29. Feel like laughing

Not at all   **Slightly**   **Moderately**   **Very much**   **Extremely**

30. Excited

Not at all   **Slightly**   **Moderately**   **Very much**   **Extremely**

31. Awe, amazement

Not at all   **Slightly**   **Moderately**   **Very much**   **Extremely**

31a. Understanding others' feelings

Not at all   **Slightly**   **Moderately**   **Very much**   **Extremely**

32. Safe

Not at all   **Slightly**   **Moderately**   **Very much**   **Extremely**

33. Feel presence of numinous force, higher power, God

Not at all   **Slightly**   **Moderately**   **Very much**   **Extremely**

34. Change in feeling about sounds in room

Not at all   **Slightly**   **Moderately**   **Very much**   **Extremely**

34a. More pleasant, less pleasant, or both

Not at all   **Slightly**   **Moderately**   **Very much**   **Extremely**

35. Happy

Not at all   **Slightly**   **Moderately**   **Very much**   **Extremely**

36. Sad

Not at all   **Slightly**   **Moderately**   **Very much**   **Extremely**

36a. Loving

Not at all   **Slightly**   **Moderately**   **Very much**   **Extremely**

37. Euphoria

Not at all   **Slightly**   **Moderately**   **Very much**   **Extremely**

38. Despair

Not at all   **Slightly**   **Moderately**   **Very much**   **Extremely**

39. Feel like crying

Not at all   **Slightly**   **Moderately**   **Very much**   **Extremely**

40. Change in feelings of closeness to people in the room

Not at all   **Slightly**   **Moderately**   **Very much**   **Extremely**

40a. Less close, closer, or both

Not at all   **Slightly**   **Moderately**   **Very much**   **Extremely**

41. Change in 'amount' of emotions

Not at all   **Slightly**   **Moderately**   **Very much**   **Extremely**

41a. Less emotional, more emotional ,or both (circle one)

42. Emotions seem different than usual

Not at all   **Slightly**   **Moderately**   **Very much**   **Extremely**

43. Feeling of oneness with the universe

Not at all   **Slightly**   **Moderately**   **Very much**   **Extremely**

44. Feel isolated from people and things

Not at all   **Slightly**   **Moderately**   **Very much**   **Extremely**

45. Feel reborn

Not at all   **Slightly**   **Moderately**   **Very much**   **Extremely**

46. Satisfaction with the experience

Not at all   **Slightly**   **Moderately**   **Very much**   **Extremely**

47. Like the experience

Not at all   **Slightly**   **Moderately**   **Very much**   **Extremely**

48. How soon would you like to repeat the experience

Never again   **Within a year**   **Within a month**   **Within a week**   **As soon as possible**

49. Desire for the experience regularly

Not at all   **Slightly**   **Moderately**   **Very much**   **Extremely**

50. An odor

Not at all   **Slightly**   **Moderately**   **Very much**   **Extremely**

50a. Please describe _____

51. A taste

Not at all   **Slightly**   **Moderately**   **Very much**   **Extremely**

51a. Please describe _____

52. A sound or sounds accompanying the experience

Not at all   **Slightly**   **Moderately**   **Very much**   **Extremely**

52a. Please describe _____

Not at all   **Slightly**   **Moderately**   **Very much**   **Extremely**

53. Sense of silence or deep quiet

Not at all   **Slightly**   **Moderately**   **Very much**   **Extremely**

54. Sounds in room sound different

Not at all   **Slightly**   **Moderately**   **Very much**   **Extremely**

55. Change in distinctiveness of sounds

Not at all   **Slightly**   **Moderately**   **Very much**   **Extremely**

55a. Less distinct, more distinct, or both (circle one)

56. Auditory synesthesia ('hearing' visual or other nonauditory perception)

Not at all   **Slightly**   **Moderately**   **Very much**   **Extremely**

57. Visual effects

Not at all   **Slightly**   **Moderately**   **Very much**   **Extremely**

58. Room looks different

Don't know   **Not**   **Slightly**   **Moderately**   **Very**   **Extremely**
eyes closed   **at all**   **much**

59. Change in brightness of objects in room

Don't know   **Not**   **Slightly**   **Moderately**   **Very**   **Extremely**
eyes closed   **at all**   **much**

59a. Brighter, duller or both (circle one)

60. Change in visual distinctness of objects in room

Don't know   **Not**   **Slightly**   **Moderately**   **Very**   **Extremely**
eyes closed   **at all**   **much**

60a. Sharper, blurrier or both (circle one)

61. Room overlaid with visual patterns

Don't know   **Not**   **Slightly**   **Moderately**   **Very**   **Extremely**
eyes closed   **at all**   **much**

62. Eyes open visual field vibrating or jiggling

Don't know   **Not**   **Slightly**   **Moderately**   **Very**   **Extremely**
eyes closed   **at all**   **much**

63. Visual synesthesia ('seeing' sound or other nonvisual perception)

Not at all   **Slightly**   **Moderately**   **Very much**   **Extremely**

64. Visual images, visions, or hallucinations (can include geometric abstract patterns)

Not at all   **Slightly**   **Moderately**   **Very much**   **Extremely**

65. Kaleidoscopic nature of images/visions/hallucinations

N/A   **Not**   **Slightly**   **Moderately**   **Very**   **Extremely**
none seen   **at all**   **much**

66. Difference in brightness of visions compared to usual daylight vision

N/A   **Not**   **Slightly**   **Moderately**   **Very**   **Extremely**
none seen   **at all**   **much**

66a. Colors brighter, duller, or both (circle one)

66b. Predominant colors_____

67. Dimensionality of images/visions/hallucinations

N/A none seen	Linear 1- dimension	Flat/planar 2- dimensions	3- dimensions	Multi- dimensions	Beyond dimensionality

68. Movement within visions/hallucinations

N/A   **Not**   **Slightly**   **Moderately**   **Very**   **Extremely**
none seen   **at all**   **much**

68a. Please describe visions/hallucinations _____

69. White light

Not at all   **Slightly**   **Moderately**   **Very much**   **Extremely**

70. Feel as if dead or dying

Not at all   **Slightly**   **Moderately**   **Very much**   **Extremely**

71. Sense of speed

Not at all   **Slightly**   **Moderately**   **Very much**   **Extremely**

72. Déjà vu (you've experienced this *exact* situation, even with no real memory of it)

Not at all   **Slightly**   **Moderately**   **Very much**   **Extremely**

73. Jamais vu (you'll experience this exact situation in the future)

Not at all   **Slightly**   **Moderately**   **Very much**   **Extremely**

74. Contradictory feelings at the same time (happy and sad; hopeful and hopeless)

Not at all   **Slightly**   **Moderately**   **Very much**   **Extremely**

75. Sense of chaos

Not at all   **Slightly**   **Moderately**   **Very much**   **Extremely**

76. Change in strength of sense of self

Not at all   **Slightly**   **Moderately**   **Very much**   **Extremely**

76a. More strongly, less strongly, or both (circle one)

77. New thoughts or insights

Not at all   **Slightly**   **Moderately**   **Very much**   **Extremely**

78. Memories of childhood

Not at all   **Slightly**   **Moderately**   **Very much**   **Extremely**

79. Feel like a child

Not at all   **Slightly**   **Moderately**   **Very much**   **Extremely**

80. Change in rate of thinking

Not at all   **Slightly**   **Moderately**   **Very much**   **Extremely**

80a. Faster, slower, or both (circle one)

81. Change in quality of thinking

Not at all   **Slightly**   **Moderately**   **Very much**   **Extremely**

81a. Sharper, duller, or both (circle one)

82. Difference in feeling of reality of experiences compared to everyday experiences

Not at all   **Slightly**   **Moderately**   **Very much**   **Extremely**

82a. Seem more real, less real, or both (circle one)

83. Dreamlike nature of the experiences

Not at all   **Slightly**   **Moderately**   **Very much**   **Extremely**

84. Thoughts of present or recent past personal life

Not at all   **Slightly**   **Moderately**   **Very much**   **Extremely**

85. Insights into personal or occupational concerns

Not at all   **Slightly**   **Moderately**   **Very much**   **Extremely**

86. Change in rate of time passing

Not at all   **Slightly**   **Moderately**   **Very much**   **Extremely**

86a. Passing faster, slower, or both (circle one)

87. Unconscious

Definitely not   **Not sure**   **Definitely Yes**

88. Change in sense of sanity

Not at all   **Slightly**   **Moderately**   **Very much**   **Extremely**

88a. More sane, less sane, or both (circle one)

89. Urge to close eyes

Not at all   **Slightly**   **Moderately**   **Very much**   **Extremely**

90. Change in effort of breathing

Not at all   **Slightly**   **Moderately**   **Very much**   **Extremely**

90a. Breathing more relaxed, more difficult, or both (circle one)

91. Able to follow the sequence of effects

Not at all   **Slightly**   **Moderately**   **Very much**   **Extremely**

92. Able to "let go"

Not at all   **Slightly**   **Moderately**   **Very much**   **Extremely**

93. Able to focus attention

Not at all   **Slightly**   **Moderately**   **Very much**   **Extremely**

94. In control

Not at all   **Slightly**   **Moderately**   **Very much**   **Extremely**

95. Able to move around if asked to do so

Not at all   **Slightly**   **Moderately**   **Very much**   **Extremely**

96. Able to remind yourself of being in a research room, being administered the drug, the temporary nature of the experience

Not at all   **Slightly**   **Moderately**   **Very much**   **Extremely**

97. Waxing and waning of the experience

Not at all   **Slightly**   **Moderately**   **Very much**   **Extremely**

98. Intensity

Not at all   **Slightly**   **Moderately**   **Very much**   **Extremely**

99. High

100. Dose you think you received

Placebo   **Dose 1 (low)**   **Dose 2**   **Dose 3**   **Dose 4 (high)**

Other comments _____

_____

_____

_____

Bibliography

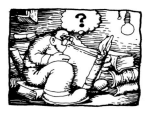

 BOOKS & DOCUMENTS

Carey, Joseph, ed. (1993). *Brain Facts: A Primer on the Brain and Nervous System.* Washington, D.C.: Society for Neuroscience.

Cerf, Christopher & Victor Navasky (1984). *The Experts Speak.* New York: Pantheon Books.

Cooper, Jack R., Floyd E. Bloom, & Robert H. Roth (1991). *The Biochemical Basis of Neuropharmacology* (6th edition). New York: Oxford University Press.

Dunnigan, James (1993). *How to Make War.* New York: Quill-William Morrow & Co.

Gans, David (1991). *Conversations with the Dead: The Grateful Dead Interview Book.* New York: Carol Publishing Group.

Hearings Before the Subcommittee on Executive Reorganization of the Committee on Government Operations (1966). U.S. Senate, 89th Congress, second session (Organization and Coordination of Federal Drug Research & Regulatory Programs: LSD) May 24-26. U.S. Government Printing Office, Washington D.C.

Hoffer, Abram & Humphrey Osmond (1967). *The Hallucinogens.* New York: Academic Press.

Hofmann, Albert (1980). *LSD: My Problem Child.* New York: McGraw Hill. Electronic version at http://www.dct.ac.uk/www/books/problem-child.html.

Kramer, Peter D. (1993). *Listening to Prozac.* New York: Penguin Books.

Leary, Denis (1992) *No Cure for Cancer.* New York: Anchor Books Doubleday.

Lee, Martin A., & Bruce Shlain (1985). *Acid Dreams: the CIA, LSD and the Sixties Rebellion.* New York: Grove Press.

Lewin, Roger (1993). *The Origin of Modern Humans.* New York: Scientific American Library.

Mader, Sylvia S. (1988). *Inquiry into Life* (5th edition). Dubuque, IA: William C. Brown Publishers.

Naranjo, Claudio (1974). *The Healing Journey: New Approaches to Consciousness.* New York: Random House.

Niven, Larry & Jerry Pournelle (1982). *Oath of Fealty.* New York: Pocket Books.

Peter, Laurence (1992). *Peter's Quotations.* New York: Quill-William Morrow.

Pletscher, A. & D. Ladewig, eds. (1994) *50 Years of LSD: Current Status and Perspectives of Hallucinogens*. New York: Parthenon Publishing Group.

Schultes, Richard E. & Albert Hofmann (1992 revised). *Plants of the Gods*. Rochester, VT: Healing Arts Press.

Shulgin, Alexander & Ann Shulgin (1991). *PIHKAL (Phenethylamines I Have Known and Loved): A Chemical Love Story*. Berkeley: Transform Press.

Siegel, Ronald, Ph.D. (1989). *Intoxication: Life in Pursuit of Artificial Paradise*. New York: E.P. Dutton.

Smith, Adam (1975). *Powers of Mind*. New York: Ballantine Books.

Smith, R. Harris (1972). *OSS: The Secret History of America's First Central Intelligence Agency*. Berkeley, CA: University of California Press.

Snyder, Solomon, M.D. (1986). *Drugs and the Brain*. New York: Scientific American Books.

Snyder, Solomon, ed. (1985). *The Encyclopedia of Psychoactive Drugs: PCP, The Dangerous Angel*. New York: Chelsea House Publishers.

Stafford, Peter (1992). *Psychedelics Encyclopedia,* 3rd expanded edition. Berkeley: Ronin Publishing.

Wallechinsky, David & Amy Wallace (1995). *The Book of Lists*. New York: Lb Books.

Watts, Alan (1989, reissue edition). *The Book on the Taboo Against Knowing Who You Are*. New York: Vintage Books.

Weil, Andrew, M.D. (1994 revised). *The Natural Mind*. New York: Houghton Mifflin.

ARTICLES

Aghajanian, George & Gerald Marek (1996). "LSD and the phenethylamine hallucinogen DOI are potent partial agonists at 5-HT$_{2A}$ receptors in rat pyriform cortex," *Journal of Pharmacology and Experimental Therapeutics*, Vol. 278:3:1373

Aghajanian, George & OHL Bing (1964). "The persistence of LSD-25 in the plasma of human subjects," *Clinical Pharmacology and Therapeutics*, Vol. 5: 611-614.

"Brain Briefings" (May 1996), Society for Neuroscience, Washington, D.C.

Clifton (popeanon@lava.net). "An interview with Alexander Shulgin," http://www.hyperreal.drugs.

Cooper, Donald (1988). "Future Synthetic Drugs Of Abuse." Drug Enforcement Administration, McLean, VA, http://www.hyperreal.com/drugs/misc.

Fackelmann, Kathy A. (Feb. 6, 1993). "Marijuana and the Brain," *Science News,* Vol. 143: 88-89.

Glennon, Richard (1991). "Introduction," *Drug Discrimination: Applications to Drug Abuse Research*. Bethesda, MD: National Institute on Drug Abuse, Department of Health and Human Services.

Glennon, Richard (1991). "Discriminative Stimulus Properties of Hallucinogens and Related Designer Drugs," *Drug Discrimination: Applications to Drug Abuse Research*, Bethesda, MD: National Institute on Drug Abuse Research Monograph Series, No. 116.

Gunn et al. (1970). "Clandestine Drug Labs," *Journal of Forensic Science*, Vol. 15:1: 51-64.

If You Change Your Mind (1994), NIH Publication No. 94-3474, produced by NIDA's Office of Science Policy, Education & Legislation.

Janiger, Oscar, M.D., & Marlene Dobkin de Rios, Ph.D. (Jan.-Mar. 1989), "LSD and Creativity," *Journal of Psychoactive Drugs*, Vol 21:1.

Kurland, Albert, Walter Pahnke, Sanford Unger, Charles Savage & Stanislov Grof (1971). "Psychedelic LSD Research," *Psychotropic Drugs in the Year 2000* (Wayne Evans, Ph.D. & Nathan Kline, M.D., eds.). Springfield, IL: Charles Thomas: 86-107.

Lotsof, H.S. (Winter 1994-95). "Ibogaine in the treatment of chemical dependence disorders: clinical perspectives," *MAPS (newsletter, Multidisciplinary Association for Psychedelic Studies)* Vol. 5:3.

LSD Use and Effects (1995). A DEA electronic article on the Internet, http://www.usdoj.gov/dea/pubs/lsd/toc.html.

MAPS Newsletter (Winter 1996-97). Vol. 7:1.

Mathias, Robert (Nov.-Dec. 1996). "The Basics of Brain Imaging," *NIDA Notes*, a publication of the National Institute on Drug Abuse, Bethesda, MD.

Mathias, Robert (March/April 1993). "NIDA Research Takes a New Look at LSD and Other Hallucinogens," *NIDA Notes*: 7-8.

NIDA Notes (Nov/Dec 1995). "Using Animals to Study Mechanisms and Effects of Drugs," National Institute on Drug Abuse, Vol. 10:6, Rockville, MD.

Shulgin, Alexander (Jan. 1976). "Profiles of Psychedelic Drugs, 1. DMT," *Journal of Psychedelic Drugs*, Vol. 8: 167-8.

Shulgin, Alexander (1987). "The Social Chemistry of Pharmacological Discovery," *Social Pharmacology*, Vol. 1: 279-290.

Szára, Stephen, M.D., D.Sc. (1968). "A Scientist Looks at the Hippies," an unpublished report to the Supervisor, Psychopharmacology Section, National Institute on Mental Health, Clinical Psychopharmacology Laboratory, St. Elizabeth's Hospital, Washington, D.C.

Strassman, Rick J, M.D. (Jan.-Mar. 1991). "Human Hallucinogenic Drug Research in the United States: A Present-Day Case History and Review of the Process," *Journal of Psychoactive Drugs,* Vol. 23: 29-38.

Strassman, Rick J., M.D. (Oct. 1984). "Adverse Reactions to Psychedelic Drugs: A Review of the Literature," *Journal of Nervous and Mental Disease*, Vol. 172:10: 578-79.

Yensen, Richard (Oct.-Dec. 1985). "LSD and Psychotherapy," *Journal of Psychoactive Drugs*, Vol. 17:4: 267-77.

 CDS

Firesign Theater (1970), from "Temporarily Humboldt County," side B (The Other Side), *Don't Crush that Dwarf, Hand Me the Pliers*, Columbia Records & Espeseth Music Music Music (ASCAP).

Steely Dan (1976). "Kid Charlemagne," by Donald Fagen & Walter Becker, from *The Royal Scam*. MCA Records, Universal City, CA.

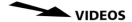 **VIDEOS**

Hofmann, Albert (1993). Videotaped message to participants at the 1993 symposium on the 50th anniversary of his discovery of LSD, April 16-17, Santa Cruz, CA, and San Francisco.

Reefer Madness (1936). Produced by George Hirliman & the FBI, directed by Louis Gasnier. Original story (*Tell Your Children*) Lawrence Meade; screenplay Arthur Hoerln; released 1985, Goodtimes Home Video Corp., NY.

Who Framed Roger Rabbit? (1988). Touchstone Pictures; Steven Spielberg & Robert Zemeckis.

The Exorcist (1973). William Friedkin, director; William Peter Blatty, screenplay. Hollywood: Warner Bros.

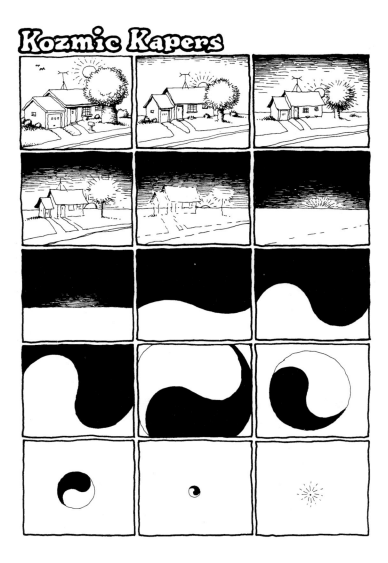

Notes

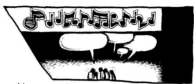

[1] *If You Change Your Mind*, NIH Publication No. 94-3474, produced by NIDA's Office of Science Policy, Education & Legislation, (1994).

[2] Laurence J. Peter, *Peter's Quotations* (New York: Quill-William Morrow, 1992): 286.

[3] Rick J. Strassman, M.D., "Hallucinogenic Drugs in Psychiatric Research and Treatment: Perspectives and Prospects," *Journal of Nervous and Mental Disease*, 1995, Vol. 183, No. 3: 127-138. These reasons are Strassman's, but other hallucinogen researchers have said similar things.

[4] Andrew Weil, M.D., *The Natural Mind,* revised (New York: Houghton-Mifflin, 1994): 44.

[5] Weil, 44-46.

[6] Weil, 45.

[7] Martin A. Lee and Bruce Shlain, *Acid Dreams: The CIA, LSD and the Sixties Rebellion* (New York: Grove Press, 1985): 90-91.

[8] Lee and Shlain, 91.

[9] Lee and Shlain, 91.

[10] Lee and Shlain, 90.

[11] Adam Smith, *Powers of Mind* (New York: Ballantine Books, 1975): 45.

[12] Richard Yensen, "Perspectives on LSD and Psychotherapy: The Search for a New Paradigm," in *50 Years of LSD: Current Status and Perspectives of Hallucinogens,* A. Pletscher and D. Ladewig, eds. Proceedings of an international symposium of the Swiss Academy of Medical Sciences, Lugano-Agno, Switzerland, Oct. 21-22, 1993 (New York: Parthenon Publishing Group, 1994): 192-194.

[13] Rick J. Strassman, "Human Hallucinogenic Drug Research in the United States: A Present-Day Case History and Review of the Process," *Journal of Psychoactive Drugs*, Vol. 23, Jan.-Mar. 1991: 29-38.

[14] Strassman, "Human Hallucinogenic Drug Research in the United States," *Journal of Psychoactive Drugs*, Jan.-Mar. 1991, Vol. 23:1: 29.

[15] Strassman, 29-38.

[16] Larry Niven and Jerry Pournelle, *Oath of Fealty* (New York: Pocket Books, 1982): 83.

[17] Ronald Siegel, *Intoxication: Life in Pursuit of Artificial Paradise* (New York: E.P. Dutton, 1989): 34-35.

[18] James Dunnigan, *How to Make War* (New York: Quill-William Morrow, 1993): 339.

[19] Siegel, 32.

[20] Laurent Rivier, "Ethnopharmacology of LSD and Related Compounds," *50 Years of LSD: Current Status and Perspectives of Hallucinogens*, A. Pletscher and D. Ladewig, eds. (New York: Parthenon Publishing Group, 1994): 43.

[21] Rivier, 43-55.

[22] Richard Yensen, "Perspectives on LSD and Psychotherapy: The Search for a New Paradigm," *50 Years of LSD* (New York: Parthenon Press, 1994): 194.

[23] Roger Lewin, *The Origin of Modern Humans* (New York: Scientific American Library, 1993): 1, 150.

[24] Rivier, 44-45.

[25] Richard E. Schultes and Albert Hofmann, *Plants of the Gods*, revised, (Rochester, VT: Healing Arts Press, 1992): 61.

[26] Richard E. Schultes and Albert Hofmann, 82-85.

[27] Rivier, 44.

[28] Richard E. Schultes and Albert Hofmann, 86.

[29] "Brain Briefings," a publication of the Society for Neuroscience, Washington, D.C., May 1996.

[30] From "The Basics of Brain Imaging" by Robert Mathias, staff writer for the Nov.-Dec. 1996 edition of *NIDA Notes*, a publication of the NIH National Institute on Drug Abuse.

[31] Isaac Asimov, Personal interview, New York City, April 1987.

[32] Solomon Snyder, M.D., *Drugs and the Brain* (New York: Scientific American Books, 1986): 7.

[33] Snyder, 26-27.

[34] Sylvia S. Mader, *Inquiry into Life*, 5th ed. (Dubuque, Iowa: William C. Brown Publishers, 1988): 320-327.

[35] Joseph Carey, ed., *Brain Facts: A Primer on the Brain and Nervous System* (Washington, D.C.: Society for Neuroscience, 1993): 4.

[36] Jack R. Cooper, Floyd E. Bloom and Robert H. Roth, *The Biochemical Basis of Neuropharmacology,* 6th ed. (New York: Oxford University Press, 1991): 11-13.

[37] Snyder, 8-9.

[38] Song title from *Lynyrd Skynyrd* by Lynyrd Skynyrd, MCI Records, (1973).

[39] Christopher Cerf and Victor Navasky, *The Experts Speak* (New York: Pantheon Books, 1984): 300.

[40] From *The Exorcist* (1973). William Friedkin, director; William Peter Blatty, screen-play. Hollywood: Warner Bros.

[41] Snyder, 207.

[42] Albert Hofmann, "History of the Discovery of LSD," in *50 Years of LSD: Current Status and Perspectives of Hallucinogens,* A. Pletscher and D. Ladewig, eds. Proceedings of an international symposium of the Swiss Academy of Medical Sciences, Lugano-Agno, Switzerland, Oct. 21-22, 1993 (New York: Parthenon Publishing Group, 1994); 13-22.

[43] Albert Hofmann, *LSD: My Problem Child* (New York: McGraw-Hill, 1980): html version @ http://www.dct.ac.uk/www/books/problem-child.html

[44] Hofmann, *LSD: My Problem Child*, html version @ http://www.dct.ac.uk/www/books/problem-child.html

[45] R. Harris Smith, *OSS: The Secret History of America's First Central Intelligence Agency* (Berkeley, CA: University of California Press, 1972): 1-10.

[46] Smith, 3.

[47] Smith, 6.

[48] Smith, 6-7.

[49] Lee and Shlain, 11.

[50] Lee and Shlain, 4-5.

[51] Smith,10, 365.

[52] Peter D. Kramer, *Listening to Prozac* (New York: Penguin Books, 1993): 327.

[53] Kramer, 327.

[54] George Aghajanian, "The Discovery of Serotonin and Its Importance to LSD Research," a presentation at the Serotonin Club dinner, 25th Annual Meeting of the Society of Neuroscience, San Diego, California, November 1995.

[55] Yensen, 195-96.

[56] Richard Yensen, "LSD and Psychotherapy," *Journal of Psychoactive Drugs*, Oct.-Dec. 1985, Vol. 17:4: 267-77.

[57] Abram Hoffer and Humphrey Osmond, *The Hallucinogens* (New York: Academic Press, 1967).

[58] Donald Cooper, *Future Synthetic Drugs Of Abuse* (McLean, VA: Drug Enforcement Administration, 1988), http://www.hyperreal.com/drugs/misc./future.html.

[59] Yensen, "Perspectives," 191-202.

[60] Lee and Shlain, 289.

[61] Lee and Shlain, 10.

[62] Lee and Shlain, 3, 11.

[63] Lee and Shlain, 10.

[64] The material in this paragraph is paraphrased and quoted from Lee and Shlain, 14-20.

[65] Lee and Shlain, 14-15.

[66] Lee and Shlain, 17.

[67] Lee and Shlain, 19.

[68] Lee and Shlain, 19.

[69] Lee and Shlain, 25.

[70] Lee and Shlain, 48-49.

71 Peter Stafford, *Psychedelics Encyclopedia*, 3rd expanded edition (Berkeley: Ronin Publishing, 1992).

72 Lee and Shlain, 24.

73 David Wallechinsky and Amy Wallace, "7 Secret CIA Mind-control Experiments," *The Book of Lists* (New York: Little Brown Books, reprint, 1995): 75-78.

74 Lee and Shlain, 30-31.

75 Wallechinsky and Wallace, 76, and Lee and Shlain, 48.

76 Wallechinsky and Wallace, 76-77.

77 Wallechinsky and Wallace, 77.

78 Wallechinsky and Wallace, 77.

79 Hofmann, "History of the Discovery of LSD," *50 Years of LSD,* 21-22.

80 Hofmann, "History of the Discovery of LSD," *50 Years of LSD*, 14.

81 Rivier, 43.

82 This paragraph is from Lee and Shlain, 57.

83 Oscar Janiger, M.D., Department of Psychiatry, University of California, Irvine, CA and Marlene Dobkin de Rios, Ph.D., Department of Anthropology, California State University, Fullerton, CA. Originally printed in the *Journal of Psychoactive Drugs*, Jan.-Mar. 1989, Vol 21: 1.

84 Lee and Shlain, 61-62.

85 Lee and Shlain, 89-90.

86 Lee and Shlain, 60-61.

87 Lee and Shlain, 60-61.

88 Lee and Shlain, 60-61.

89 Laurence J. Peter, 260.

90 Hanscarl Leuner (1918-1996), a pioneer of hallucinogen research and psycholytic therapy, "Hallucinogens as an Aid in Psychotherapy: Basic Principles and Results," *50 Years of LSD,* 175-189.

91 Lee and Shlain, 150.

92 Smith, 45.

93 Albert Kurland, Walter Pahnke, Sanford Unger, Charles Savage, and Stanislov Grof, "Psychedelic LSD Research," *Psychotropic Drugs in the Year 2000*, eds. Wayne Evans, Ph.D., and Nathan Kline, M.D. (Springfield, Illinois: Charles Thomas, 1971): 86-107.

94 From Stephen Szára, M.D., D.Sc., "A Scientist Looks at the Hippies," (Washington, D.C., 1968). Used with permission.

95 U.S. Senate, 89th Congress, second session, Organization and Coordination of Federal Drug Research & Regulatory Programs: LSD, *Hearings Before the Subcommittee on Executive Reorganization of the Committee on Government Operations* (Washington, D.C.: U.S. Government Printing Office, May 24-26, 1966).

96 Lee and Shlain, xx-xxi.

97 Denis Leary, *No Cure for Cancer* (New York: Anchor Books, Doubleday, 1992): 54.

[98] "Using Animals to Study Mechanisms and Effects of Drugs," *NIDA Notes* (Rockville, Maryland: National Institute on Drug Abuse, Nov.-Dec. 1995, Vol. 10:6): SR-3, SR-4.

[99] Richard Glennon, "Introduction," *Drug Discrimination: Applications to Drug Abuse Research* (Bethesda: National Institute on Drug Abuse, Research Monograph Series, No. 116, 1991): 1.

[100] Richard Glennon, "Discriminative Stimulus Properties of Hallucinogens and Related Designer Drugs," in *Drug Discrimination: Applications to Drug Abuse Research* (Bethesda: National Institute on Drug Abuse, Research Monograph Series, No. 116, 1991): 25.

[101] "The Social Chemistry of Discovery: The DMT Story," in *Social Pharmacology*, 1989, 3(3): 237-248.

[102] Firesign Theater, "Temporarily Humboldt County," side B (The Other Side) on *Don't Crush that Dwarf, Hand Me the Pliers*, from Columbia Records & Espeseth Music Music Music (ASCAP), 1970.

[103] Rick J. Strassman, M.D., "Human Psychopharmacology of LSD," *50 Years of LSD*, 157.

[104] Firesign Theater, "Temporarily Humboldt County," side B (The Other Side) on *Don't Crush that Dwarf, Hand Me the Pliers*.

[105] Snyder, 164-177.

[106] Snyder, 170-171.

[107] Kathy A. Fackelmann, "Marijuana and the Brain," *Science News*, Feb. 6, 1993, Vol. 143: 88-89.

[108] Robert Mathias, "NIDA Research Takes a New Look at LSD and Other Hallucinogens," *NIDA Notes*, Rockville, Maryland: National Institute on Drug Abuse, March-April 1993: 7-8.

[109] Albert Hofmann, from the transcript of a videotaped message to participants at a 1993 symposium held April 16 in Santa Cruz, California, and April 17 in San Francisco on the 50th anniversary of his discovery of LSD.

[110] Dieter Ladewig, "Conclusions," *50 Years of LSD*, 223-228.

[111] Rick Strassman, M.D., "Adverse Reactions to Psychedelic Drugs: A Review of the Literature," *Journal of Nervous and Mental Disease*, Oct. 1984, Vol. 172: 10: 578-579.

[112] Adolf Dittrich, "Psychological Aspects of Altered States of Consciousness of the LSD Type: Measuring Basic Dimensions and Predicting Individual Differences," *50 Years of LSD*, 101-118.

[113] George Aghajanian and OHL Bing, "The Persistence of LSD-25 in the Plasma of Human Subjects," *Clinical Pharmacology and Therapeutics*, 1964, Vol. 5: 611-614.

[114] George Aghajanian & Gerald Marek "LSD and the Phenethylamine Hallucinogen DOI are Potent Partial Agonists at $5\text{-}HT_{2A}$ Receptors on Interneurons in Rat Pyriform Cortex," *Journal of Pharmacology and Experimental Therapeutics*, 1996, Vol. 278:3:1373

[115] Snyder, 16.

[116] Joseph Carey, ed., *Brain Facts: A Primer on the Brain and Nervous System* (Washington, D.C.: Society for Neuroscience, 1993): 32.

[117] Richard E. Schultes and Albert Hofmann, 122-123.

[118] Rivier, 47.

[119] Schultes and Hofmann, 160-62.

[120] Schultes and Hofmann, 132-143.

[121] Hofmann, *LSD: My Problem Child,* html version @ http://www.dct.ac.uk/www/books/problem-child.html.

[122] Hofmann, "History of the Discovery of LSD,"*50 Years of LSD:* 13-14.

[123] Alexander Shulgin, "Profiles of Psychedelic Drugs. 1. DMT," *Psychedelic Drugs*, 1976, 8: 167-168.

[124] Schultes and Hofmann, 112-115.

[125] Mark Molliver and Elizabeth O'Hearn, "Ibogaine Neurotoxicity Raises New Questions in Addiction Research," *Journal of NIH Research*, November 1993, Vol. 5: 11: 50-55.

[126] From the U.S. Patent and Trademark Office Web site at http://www.uspto.gov.

[127] H.S. Lotsof, "Ibogaine in the Treatment of Chemical Dependence Disorders: Clinical Perspectives," *MAPS newsletter*, Winter 1994-95, Vol. 5: 3.

[128] Alexander Shulgin and Ann Shulgin, *PIHKAL: (Phenethylamines I Have Known and Loved): A Chemical Love Story* (Berkeley: Transform Press, 1991), html version at http://www.hyperreal.com/drugs/pihkal/index.html.

[129] Shulgin and Shulgin, html version.

[130] Shulgin and Shulgin, html version.

[131] Shulgin and Shulgin, html version.

[132] Eugeny Krupitsky, M.D., Ph.D., and A.M. Burakov, M.D., "Continued Studies into Underlying Psychological Mechanisms of Ketamine Psychedelic Therapy," *MAPS,* Spring 1996,Vol. 1: 3.

[133] Solomon Snyder, M.D., ed., *The Encyclopedia of Psychoactive Drugs: PCP, The Dangerous Angel* (New York: Chelsea House Publishers, 1985): 19-43.

[134] Shulgin and Shulgin, html version.

[135] Lee and Shlain, 37-38.

[136] Claudio Naranjo, *The Healing Journey* (New York: Random House, 1974).

[137] David Nichols, professor of medicinal chemistry and pharmacology, Purdue, personal communication, April 1997.

[138] Shulgin and Shulgin, html version.

[139] David Nichols, "Differences Between the Mechanism of Action of MDMA, MDB, and the Classic Hallucinogens," *Journal of Psychoactive Drugs*, 1986, Vol. 18: 305-313.

[140] Nicholas Saunders, "E Is for Ecstasy," on-line at http://www.hyperreal.com/drugs/e4x.

[141] Clifton [popeanon@lava.net], electronic article at http://www.hyperreal.com/drugs.

[142] Shulgin and Shulgin, html version.

[143] Clifton (Shulgin interview), http://www.hyperreal.com/drugs.

144 Produced by George A. Hirliman in collaboration with the FBI, directed by Louis Gasnier. Original story (*Tell Your Children*) by Lawrence Meade, screenplay by Arthur Hoerl, additional dialogue by Paul Franklin, *Reefer Madness,* B&W, 67 min., released 1985 by Goodtimes Home Video Corp., New York, 1936.

145 From the National Organization for the Reform of Marijuana Laws (NORML-est 1970) home page @ http://www.norml.org/norml/.

146 Lee and Shlain, 146-147.

147 David Gans, *Conversations with the Dead: The Grateful Dead Interview Book* (New York: Carol Publishing Group, 1991): 310.

148 Gans, 309.

149 Gans, 322-323.

150 Gunn et al., "Clandestine Drug Labs," *Journal of Forensic Science*, 1970, Vol. 15:1: 51-64.

151 Gunn et al., 63-64.

152 Weil, 45.

153 MAPS newsletter, Vol. 7:1, Winter 1996-1997. The article is on-line in the newsletter at http://www.maps.org.

154 Alan Watts, *The Book: On the Taboo Against Knowing Who You Are*, reissue edition, New York: Vintage Books, 1989: 32.

155 From "Vignettes: Comforts of Science," *Science*, Vol. 270, Dec. 22, 1995. Originally from Linus Pauling as quoted in *Linus Pauling in His Own Words*. Barbara Marinacci, ed., Simon & Schuster, 1951.

156 Rick J. Strassman, M.D., "Hallucinogen Rating Scale," ©1994. Used with permission.

Index

195, 197-198, 200, 211, 214, 218-219, 239-248

"LSD and Chromosomes: A Controlled Experiment," xxii

LSD effects, 48, 82, 110, 118

LSD outpatient therapy, 176

LSD psychoses, 108

LSD: My Problem Child, 34, 107, 214, 239, 242, 245, 248

Lugano-Agno, Switzerland, xi, 243, 245

lymphocytes, xx-xxi, 170

lysergic acid amide [ergine], 129

lysergic acid amide, 58, 129

lysergic acid butanolamide, 34

lysergic acid diethylamide *see* LSD

lysergic acid hydroethylamide, 129

lysergic acid hydroxyethylamide, 58

lysergic acid propanolamide, 34

lysergic acid, 34-35, 58-59, 84, 129

lysergsäure-diäthylamid, 34

magic, 14, 58, 77, 107, 139, 164, 218

magnet, 18

magnetic fields, 38

magnetic resonance imaging (MRI), 16-19, 97

magnetic resonance spectroscopy, 149

malignant hyperthermic response, 150

Manaus, Brazil, 127

MAO Inhibitors, 120, 124, 195

MAPS *see* Multidisciplinary Association for Psychedelic Studies

Marijuana Tax Act of 1937, 5, 77

marijuana use among teenagers, xvi, 224

marijuana, xiii, xvi, 5, 31, 38, 64, 72, 75, 77-78, 90, 109, 156-159, 163-164, 170, 174,

181, 184-185, 214, 216, 218-219, 224, 228, 240, 247, 249

Maryland Psychiatric Research Center, 73

Mash, Deborah, 178

matched controls, 127

Mazatec Indians, 58

McGill University, 55

McKenna, Dennis, 127, 178-179

MDA, xx, 5, 82-83, 85, 113, 141-142, 144-146, 180

MDE, 113, 141, 177, 180

MDMA, xx, 7, 83, 85, 113-114, 123-124, 141-153, 164-165, 167, 170, 175-176, 180-181, 195, 197, 219, 228, 248 *see also* ecstasy

MDMA-assisted psychotherapy, 175

Mechoulam, Raphael, 91

Medical College of Virginia School of Pharmacy, 81, 152

medical arguments against LSD, xxii

medical ethics, 43, 53

medical marijuana, 174, 181, 184-185, 214

medical utility, 6

medicinal chemistry, 81, 111, 152, 248

medicinal chemists, x, xvii

meditation, 64, 74, 228

Medline database, 180

medulla oblongata, 22

melatonin, 7

memories, 44, 106, 114, 236

memory blocks, 44

mental equilibrium, 119

mental health, 68, 168-169, 171, 194, 215, 220, 224-225, 241

mental illness, 39, 108, 219

mental problems, xix, 97

Merck, 142

mescal buttons, 130

mescaline, xx, 5, 45, 50, 56, 60, 64, 82, 84-87, 95, 97, 106, 111-113, 117, 119, 127, 130, 137-139, 141-142, 175, 179-180, 197-198, 213, 224

Mesolithic Age, 14

metabolism, 19, 21, 24, 39, 57, 67, 97, 120, 128, 181

metabolite, 71, 120, 131-132, 137

methamphetamine, 85, 113, 177

Methergine, 34

methyl group, 82, 85, 137

Metzner, Ralph, 0, 149, 227, 229

midbrain, 22

Middle Ages, 33

midwives, 33

migrant nomads, 14

military intelligence, 52

mind control, 38, 50, 246

mind-blowing drugs, xx

mint, 178

misinformation, 73, 98, 200, 225

mistrust, 198

MK-ULTRA, 53

molecular pharmacologists, xvii

molecular pharmacology, xvii, 111

Molliver, Mark, 135, 144, 164, 248

monoamine oxidase inhibitors, 120, 122, 195

mood disorders, xvii, 110

mood regulation, 148

mood, xvii, xix, xxv, 3, 13, 23-24, 44, 96, 106, 110-111, 115, 118-119, 131, 148, 151, 188, 195-196

morning glory seeds, 106, 128

morning glory, 58, 106, 128-129

morphine, 13, 26, 50, 57, 90, 151, 156

motor nerves, 19-20

Mount Pinatubo, 198

MRI *see* magnetic resonance imaging

Multidisciplinary Association for Psychedelic Studies (MAPS), 122, 173-174, 180, 218-219, 241, 248-249

multiple personality disorder, 183

mushroom cult, 58

mushrooms, xxiv, 15, 58, 77-78, 128, 130-131, 218

sacred mushrooms, 128, 130
sacred plants, 5
Sahara Desert, 15
saline solution, 80
Salvia divinorum, 178
Salvinorin A, 178
San Francisco, 43, 72, 74, 76, 174, 179, 186-187, 211, 217, 242, 247
San Pedro de Acatama, 15
Sandoz, 13, 15, 33-34, 36, 44, 60-61, 75, 98-99, 187, 214
Sanskrit, 92
Saskatchewan, Canada, 45
Satan, 31
Saturday Evening Post, 73
Schaefer, Stacy, 178
Schedule I, 6, 142-144, 156-161, 171, 184
scheduling criteria, 158
schizophrenia, xviii-xix, 3, 23, 25, 45-46, 49, 100, 106, 115, 197
scientific base, 100
Scully, Tim, 187
Seconal, 91, 133
secret research, 43
selective serotonin reup-take inhibitor (SSRI), 120, 124
Senate subcommittee on executive reorganization, 69
sensory deprivation, 38, 55, 110, 228
sensory information, 115
sensory output, 22
sensory overload, 110
separate realities, 111
serotonergic, 55-56, 120, 151, 164, 176-177
Serotonin Club, 56, 114, 245
serotonin biochemistry, 128
serotonin deficiency, 147-148
serotonin release, 85, 145-146
serotonin, xii, 13, 23-25, 28, 38-40, 48, 55-57, 67-68, 71, 83, 85, 113-121, 124, 128-129, 131-132, 142-143, 145-149, 151-152, 164, 170, 177,
179, 192-193, 195-196, 245
sertraline, 120, 123
Serturner, Friedrich, 13
set and setting, 97, 128, 188
sexual aberrations, 40
sexual effect, 94
sexual psychopaths, 54
Shalala, Donna, xvi
shaman, 14, 187-188
Shaw, George Bernard, xiv
Shelley, Mary Wollstonecraft, 19
Shulgin, Alexander and Ann, 139, 224, 248
Siberia, 14
Siegel, Dr. Ron, 11
single-photon-emission computed tomography (SPECT), 17-18, 149
sites of action, 28, 97, 145, 177
sleep, 24, 38, 46, 55, 122, 131, 135, 196, 228-229
Smith, Dr. Bob, 48
Smith, R. Harris, 37, 240, 245
Smithsonian Institution, 30
Smythies, John, 45
snuff powders, 59-60
Snyder, Solomon, 24, 31, 57, 69, 240, 244, 248
social movements, 5
socialize, 199
Society for Neuroscience, xxiii, 221, 239-240, 244, 247
Society for the Investigation of Human Ecology, 55
sodium pentothal, 44
Soma, 14
South America, 0, 43, 59, 85, 125, 188
South American Indians, 15, 59-60, 181
SPECT *see* single-photon-emission computed tomography
speech-inducing sub-stance, 50
speed, 33, 48, 75, 78, 106, 194, 227, 229, 231, 233, 235-237
spinal tap, 31, 120
spirit world, 14, 125, 134
spiritual beliefs, 199
spiritual states, 106
Spring Grove State Hospital, 68
SSRI *see* selective sero-tonin reuptake inhibitor
St. Anthony's Fire, 33
St. Elizabeth's Hospital, 73, 75, 241
Stanley, Augustus Owsley, 11, 187
stimulant, 82-83, 85, 133, 144, 152
stimulation, 38, 124, 133, 135
Stoll, Arthur, 33
straight line, 52, 107
Strassman, Rick, 7-8, 89, 93, 95, 97, 99, 107, 170-171, 181, 192, 227, 230, 241, 247
street drugs, 156, 186-187, 190-191, 194, 197, 199
stress, 52, 106, 140, 151, 182
structure, 17, 34, 49, 80, 91, 112, 114, 129-131, 156, 192
strychnine, 13
subjective emotions, 92
substance abuse, 149, 168, 182, 208-210, 216, 220-221, 223-224
substance use, 198, 208-209
substituted phenethy-lamines, 139
suicidal thoughts, xvii
suicide, 5, 54, 110
Summer of Love, 5, 98, 162, 166
Sunset Strip, 74
surgeon general, 11
survey results, 198
Swiss Academy of Medical Sciences, 98-99, 243, 245
sympathetic nerves, 25, 196
synapse, 20, 23-24, 29-30, 120, 146
synaptic gaps, 20, 22, 27
synaptic vesicles, 25, 28
synesthesia, 106, 111, 234-235
synthetic heroin, 143, 191
Szára, Stephen, 59, 72-73, 75, 86, 133, 173, 241, 246

Picture Credits